iDEALHEALTH'S
# PLANT-BASED DIET FOR WEIGHT LOSS

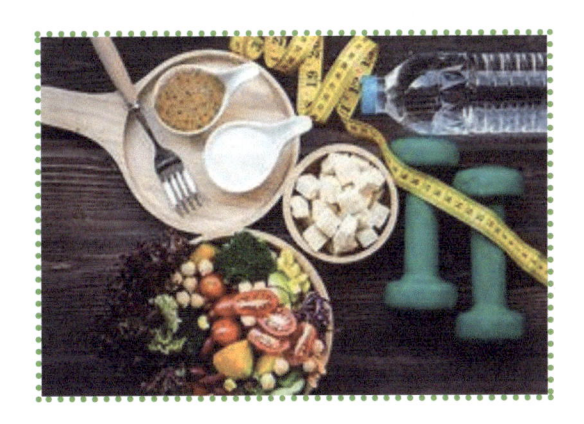

A Simple and Effective Guide to Eat Plants and Lose Weight.

## Author's Love Note

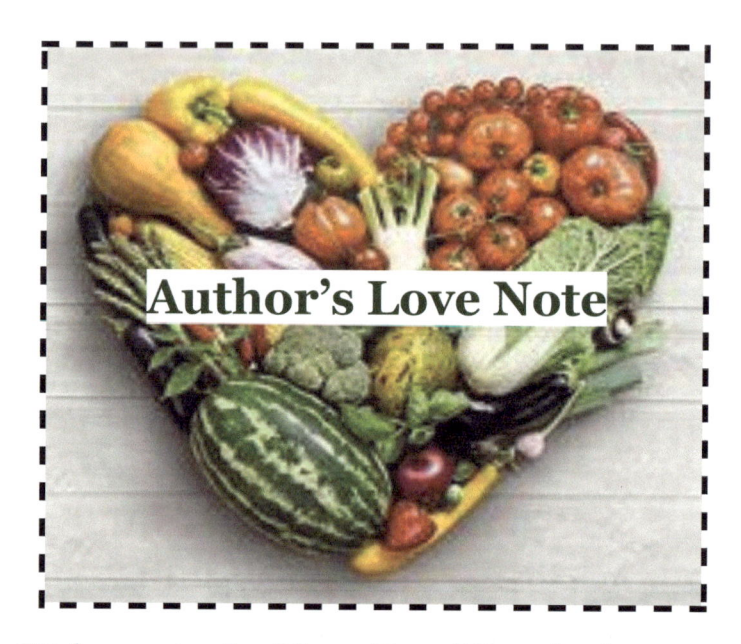

**Welcome to the Plant-Based Revolution!**

Are you tired of feeling sluggish, weighed down, and stuck in a cycle of unhealthy eating? Do you dream of a vibrant, energetic, and radiant you, with a body that thrives on whole, plant-based foods? You're not alone!

In recent years, the world has witnessed a profound shift in how we think about food, health, and wellness. The plant-based revolution has taken center stage, with millions of people around the globe embracing a lifestyle that celebrates the incredible benefits of whole, plant-based foods.

**A Journey of Transformation**

This book is your invitation to join the plant-based revolution and embark on a transformative journey that will change how you think about food, your body, and your health. Within these pages, you'll discover the incredible power of plant-based eating to:

- Boost your energy and vitality
- Support a healthy weight and body composition
- Enhance your mental clarity and focus
- Nurture a strong and resilient immune system
- Cultivate a deeper connection with your body and the natural world

**A Comprehensive Guide**

"Plant-Based Diet for Weight Loss" is more than just a cookbook or a diet plan-it's a comprehensive guide to embracing a plant-based lifestyle that will support your overall health, wellness, and weight loss goals. Inside, you'll find:

- → A clear and concise introduction to the benefits of plant-based eating
- → A simple and effective 7-day meal plan to get you started
- → Over 50 delicious and easy-to-make plant-based recipes
- → Practical tips and strategies for meal planning, grocery shopping, and eating out
- → Expert advice on overcoming common obstacles and staying on track

**Join the Movement**

So, if you're ready to join the plant-based revolution and start your journey towards a healthier, happier, and more vibrant you, this book is for you!

**Let's get started on this incredible journey together! See you on the inside!**

# Table of Content

Introduction

The Benefits of Plant-Based Eating for Weight Loss and Optimal Health.

How to Use This Book: Unlocking the Secrets to a Vibrant, Plant-Based Lifestyle

Part 1: The Science of Plant-Based Eating

Chapter 1: The Power of Plant-Based Nutrition

Chapter 2: Debunking Common Myths About Plant-Based Diets

Chapter 3: The Benefits of Plant-Based Eating for Weight Loss and Overall Health

Part 2: Getting Started with Plant-Based Eating

Chapter 4: Setting Up Your Plant-Based Kitchen

Chapter 5: Stocking Your Pantry with Plant-Based Essentials

Chapter 6: Meal Planning and Grocery Shopping for Plant-Based Success

Part 3: Delicious Plant-Based Recipes for Weight Loss

Chapter 7: Breakfast Recipes for a Plant-Based Boost

Chapter 8: Lunch and Dinner Recipes for a Plant-Based Lifestyle

Chapter 9: Snacks and Desserts for a Guilt-Free Treat

Part 4: Overcoming Common Obstacles and Staying on Track

Chapter 10: Common Challenges and Solutions for Plant-Based Eaters

Chapter 11: Staying Motivated and Accountable on Your Plant-Based Journey

Chapter 12: Navigating Social Situations and Eating Out on a Plant-Based Diet

Part 5: Putting it All Together for Lasting Success

Chapter 13: Part 5: Putting it All Together for Lasting Success

Chapter 14: Mindful Eating and Self-Care for a Healthy Relationship with Food
Chapter 15: Maintaining Momentum and Celebrating Your Successes

Conclusion
Congratulations on Completing the Plant-Based Diet for Weight Loss Journey!
Next Steps and Continued Support

Appendix
Plant-Based Resources and Recommendations
Meal Planning Templates and Worksheets
Plant-Based Nutrition Glossary

# Introduction

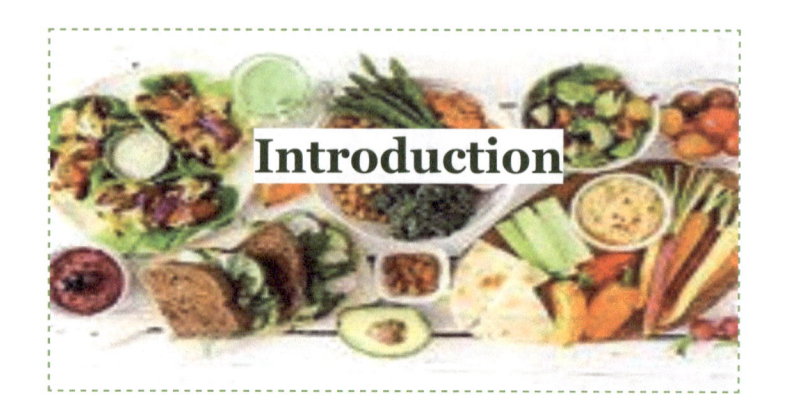

**Welcome to the Plant-Based Revolution!**

Imagine a world where vibrant health, boundless energy, and radiant well-being are the norm. A world where the air is clean, the oceans are thriving, and the land is fertile. A world where food is not just sustenance, but a powerful tool for transformation.

This revolution is not just about food; it's about a way of life. It's about choosing compassion over cruelty, sustainability over destruction, and vitality over stagnation. It's about joining a global movement that's redefining the way we eat, live, and interact with the world around us.

**The Power of Plant-Based Eating**

For decades, we've been told that a healthy diet requires animal products. We've been led to believe that meat, dairy, and eggs are essential for strong bones, robust health, and peak performance. But the truth is, a plant-based diet is not only sufficient; it's superior.

Plant-based eating has been shown to:

- ❖ Reduce the risk of chronic diseases like heart disease, diabetes, and certain types of cancer
- ❖ Promote weight loss and improve body composition
- ❖ Boost energy levels and enhance mental clarity
- ❖ Support healthy digestion and reduce inflammation
- ❖ Nurture a strong and resilient immune system

**Join the Movement**

The plant-based revolution is not just about individual transformation; it's about collective impact. It's about creating a world where:

- Animals are treated with respect, kindness, and compassion
- The environment is protected, preserved, and restored
- Food is produced, distributed, and consumed in a way that's fair, just, and sustainable

**What to Expect**

In the following pages, we'll take you on a journey of discovery, exploration, and transformation. We'll share with you:

- The science behind plant-based eating and its numerous health benefits
- Practical tips and strategies for transitioning to a plant-based lifestyle

- Delicious, easy-to-make recipes that will inspire and delight you
- Expert advice on overcoming common obstacles and staying on track
- Inspiring stories of people who've transformed their lives with plant-based eating

**Get Ready to Transform Your Life!**

The plant-based revolution is not just a diet; it's a way of life. It's a choice to live with intention, compassion, and purpose. It's a decision to take control of your health, well-being, and impact on the world.

So, if you're ready to join the revolution, if you're ready to transform your life, and if you're ready to make a difference, then let's get started!

Together, we can create a world that's healthier, happier, and more sustainable for all.

## *The Benefits of Plant-Based Eating for Weight Loss and Optimal Health. Unlock the Power of Plant-Based Eating for Weight Loss and Optimal Health*

Are you tired of feeling sluggish, weighed down, and stuck in a cycle of unhealthy eating? Do you dream of a vibrant, energetic, and radiant you, with a body that thrives on whole, plant-based foods? You're not alone!

Plant-based eating has been shown to have numerous benefits for weight loss and optimal health. From boosting your energy levels and enhancing your mental clarity to supporting a healthy weight and body composition, and reducing the risk of chronic diseases, plant-based eating is the key to unlocking your full potential.

**Weight Loss Benefits**
1. Lower Calorie Intake: Plant-based foods tend to be lower in calories and higher in fiber, making it easier to maintain a healthy weight.
2. Increased Satiety: Plant-based foods are rich in fiber, which helps keep you feeling fuller for longer, reducing the likelihood of overeating.
3. Improved Gut Health: A plant-based diet is rich in prebiotic fiber, which helps feed the good bacteria in your gut, supporting a healthy gut microbiome.
4. Reduced Inflammation: Plant-based foods are rich in antioxidants and polyphenols, which help reduce inflammation and promote overall health.

**Optimal Health Benefits**
1. Reduced Risk of Chronic Diseases: Plant-based eating has been shown to reduce the risk of heart disease, type 2 diabetes, and certain types of cancer.
2. Improved Heart Health: Plant-based foods are rich in healthy fats, fiber, and antioxidants, which help support heart health and reduce the risk of cardiovascular disease.
3. Enhanced Mental Clarity and Focus: Plant-based foods are rich in omega-3 fatty acids, vitamins, and minerals, which help support brain health and enhance mental clarity and focus.
4. Stronger Immune System: Plant-based foods are rich in antioxidants, vitamins, and minerals, which help support immune function and reduce the risk of illness and disease.

**Additional Benefits**
1. Increased Energy: Plant-based foods are rich in iron, vitamin B12, and other essential nutrients, which help support energy production and reduce fatigue.
2. Improved Digestion: Plant-based foods are rich in fiber, which helps promote regular bowel movements, prevent constipation, and support healthy digestion.
3. Glowing Skin: Plant-based foods are rich in antioxidants, vitamins, and minerals, which help support skin health and reduce the signs of aging.
4. Reduced Environmental Impact: Animal agriculture is a leading cause of greenhouse gas emissions, deforestation, and water pollution. Plant-based eating is a powerful way to reduce your environmental footprint.

**Getting Started**
1. Start with Small Changes: Begin by incorporating more plant-based meals into

your diet and gradually reduce your intake of animal products.
2. Explore New Foods: Try new fruits, vegetables, whole grains, and legumes to find healthy, plant-based options that you enjoy.
3. Seek Out Support: Connect with friends, family, or a healthcare professional who can support and guide you on your plant-based journey.
4. Be Patient and Kind to Yourself: Remember that transitioning to a plant-based lifestyle takes time, patience, and self-compassion. Be gentle with yourself, and don't be afraid to make mistakes.

Plant-based eating will help you unlock the door to a vibrant, energetic, and radiant you. So you shouldn't hesitate to start your plant-based journey to discover the incredible benefits that await you!

# How to Use This Book: Unlocking the Secrets to a Vibrant, Plant-Based Lifestyle

Congratulations on taking the first step towards transforming your health, wellbeing, and relationship with food! This book is your comprehensive guide to embracing a plant-based lifestyle, and we're excited to share this journey with you.

**A Personalized Approach**

This book is designed to be a personalized guide, tailored to your unique needs, goals, and preferences. Whether you're a beginner, intermediate, or advanced plant-based enthusiast, you'll find valuable insights, practical tips, and delicious recipes to support your journey.

**Navigating the Book**

To get the most out of this book, we recommend the following:

1. Start with the Introduction: Get familiar with the benefits of plant-based eating, and understand the philosophy behind this lifestyle.
2. Explore the Chapters: Dive into the chapters that resonate with you the most, whether it's learning about the science behind plant-based eating, exploring delicious recipes, or overcoming common obstacles.
3. Take Notes and Reflect: As you read through the book, take notes on the insights, tips, and recipes that resonate with you. Reflect on your progress, and celebrate your successes.
4. Try New Recipes: Get cooking with our delicious, easy-to-make recipes! Experiment with new flavors, ingredients, and techniques to find your favorite plant-based dishes.

5. Join the Community: Connect with like-minded individuals who share your passion for plant-based living. Join online communities, attend local events, and participate in discussions to expand your knowledge and support network.

**Customizing Your Experience**

To tailor this book to your unique needs, consider the following:

1. Identify Your Goals: What do you want to achieve through plant-based eating? Is it weight loss, improved health, or environmental sustainability? Focus on the chapters and recipes that align with your goals.
2. Assess Your Lifestyle: Consider your lifestyle, including your schedule, budget, and cooking skills. Choose recipes and tips that fit your reality, and don't be afraid to adapt or modify them as needed.

3. Explore New Ingredients: Venture out of your comfort zone and try new ingredients, flavors, and cuisines. This will help you stay engaged, motivated, and inspired on your plant-based journey.

**A Journey, Not a Destination**

Remember, embracing a plant-based lifestyle is a journey, not a destination. It's a process of growth, exploration, and self-discovery. Be patient, kind, and compassionate with yourself as you navigate this journey.

**Let's Get Started!**

You're now ready to embark on this transformative journey. Take a deep breath, turn the page, and let's dive into the world of plant-based eating together!

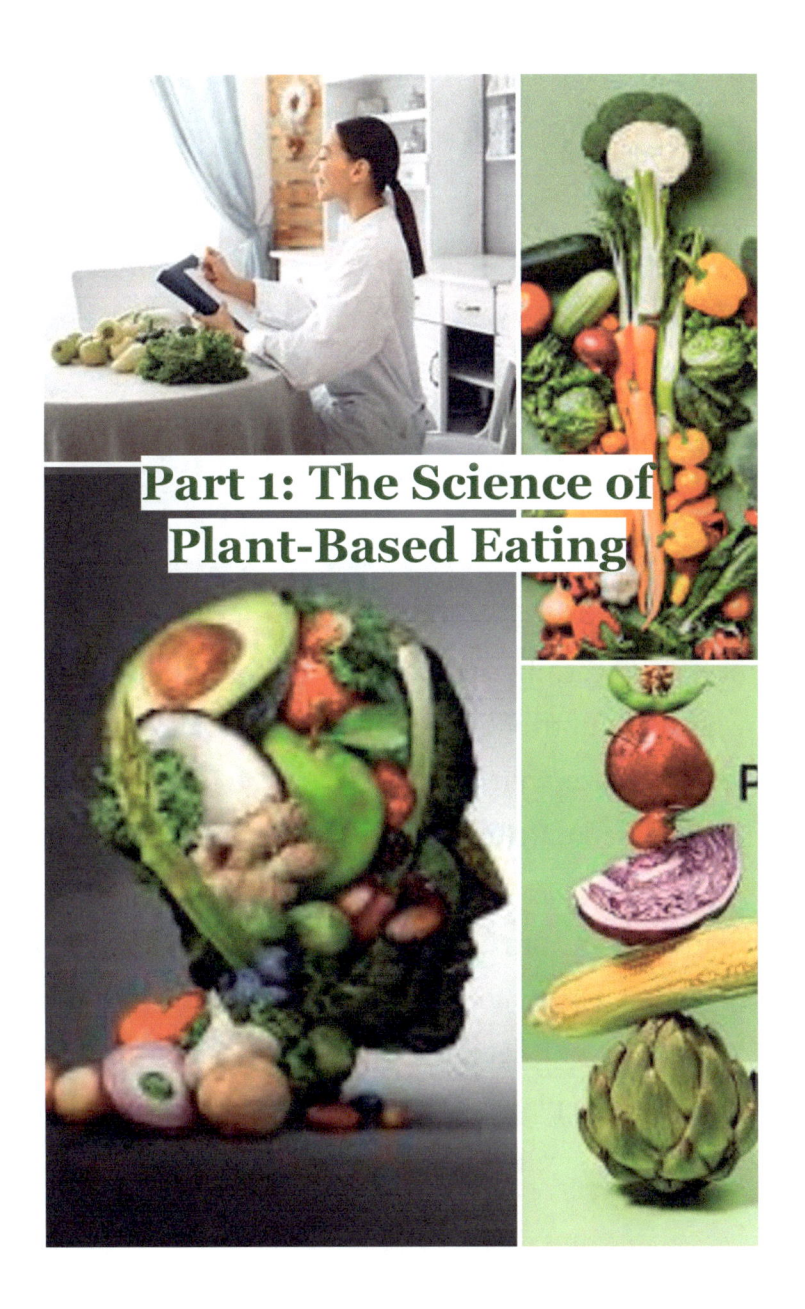

# Part 1: The Science of Plant-Based Eating

## Chapter 1:

## The Power of Plant-Based Nutrition: Unlocking the Secrets to Optimal Health

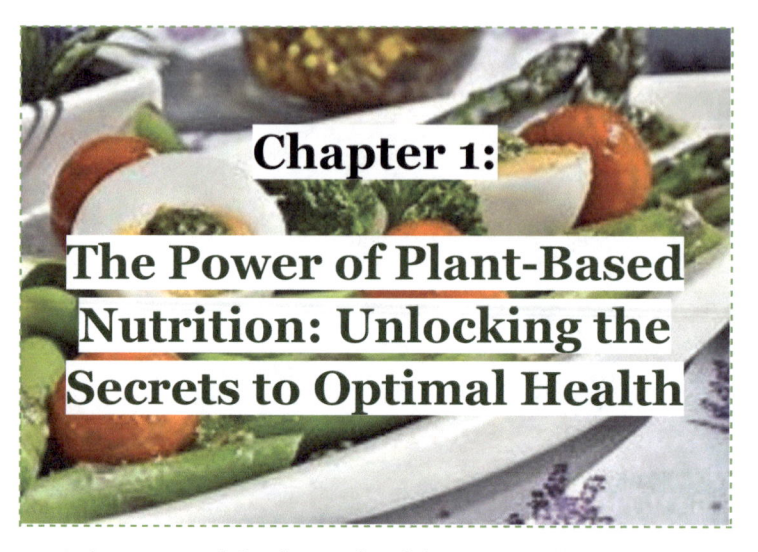

Imagine a world where food is not just sustenance, but a powerful tool for transformation. A world where the nutrients you consume can heal, protect, and energize your body. Welcome to the world of plant-based nutrition!

Plant-based nutrition is not just a diet; it's a lifestyle. It's a choice to fuel your body with the most nutrient-dense, vibrant, and life-affirming foods on the planet. It's a decision to take control of your health, well-being, and destiny.

## The Science Behind Plant-Based Nutrition

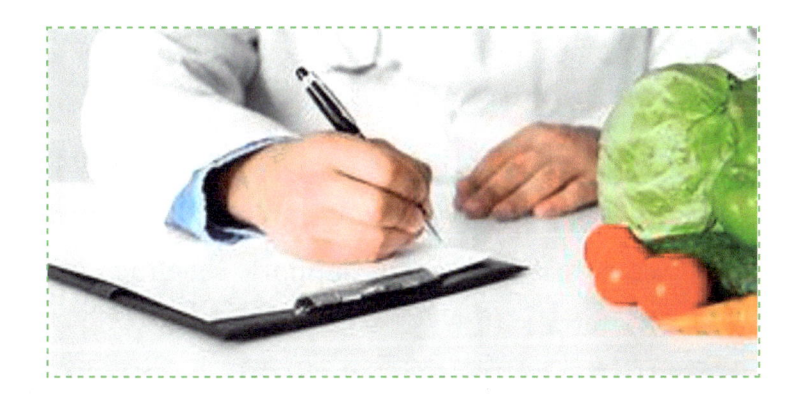

Plant-based foods are packed with an array of vitamins, minerals, antioxidants, and phytochemicals that work synergistically to promote optimal health. These nutrients have been shown to:

1. Boost Immune Function: Plant-based foods are rich in vitamin C, vitamin E, and beta-carotene, which help support immune function and protect against illness and disease.
2. Reduce Inflammation: Plant-based foods are rich in anti-inflammatory compounds like

omega-3 fatty acids, antioxidants, and polyphenols, which help reduce inflammation and promote healing.
3. Support Healthy Digestion: Plant-based foods are rich in fiber, which helps promote regular bowel movements, prevent constipation, and support healthy gut bacteria.
4. Protect Against Chronic Diseases: Plant-based foods have been shown to reduce the risk of chronic diseases like heart disease, type 2 diabetes, and certain types of cancer.

**The Benefits of Plant-Based Nutrition**

The benefits of plant-based nutrition are numerous and well-documented. By incorporating more plant-based foods into your diet, you can:

1. Lose Weight and Improve Body Composition: Plant-based foods are generally lower in calories and higher in

fiber, making it easier to maintain a healthy weight and body composition.
2. Improve Mental Clarity and Focus: Plant-based foods are rich in antioxidants, vitamins, and minerals that help support brain health and improve mental clarity and focus.
3. Boost Energy and Vitality: Plant-based foods are rich in iron, vitamin B12, and other essential nutrients that help support energy production and reduce fatigue.
4. Support Healthy Skin, Hair, and Nails: Plant-based foods are rich in antioxidants, vitamins, and minerals that help support healthy skin, hair, and nails.

## The Best Plant-Based Foods for Optimal Health

While all plant-based foods offer nutritional benefits, some stand out for their exceptional nutritional value. These include:

1. Leafy Greens: Spinach, kale, collard greens, and other leafy greens are rich in vitamins A, C, and K, as well as minerals like calcium and iron.
2. Berries: Blueberries, strawberries, raspberries, and other berries are rich in antioxidants, vitamins C and K, and minerals like manganese and copper.
3. Legumes: Lentils, chickpeas, black beans, and other legumes are rich in protein, fiber, and minerals like potassium, magnesium, and iron.
4. Nuts and Seeds: Almonds, walnuts, chia seeds, and other nuts and seeds are rich in healthy fats, protein, and minerals like magnesium, potassium, and zinc.

## Incorporating Plant-Based Nutrition into Your Lifestyle

Incorporating plant-based nutrition into your lifestyle is easier than you think! Here are some simple tips to get you started:

1. Start with Small Changes: Begin by incorporating one or two plant-based meals into your diet each day.
2. Explore New Recipes: Try new plant-based recipes and flavors to keep your diet interesting and varied.
3. Shop Smart: Stock your pantry and fridge with a variety of plant-based foods, including fruits, vegetables, whole grains, and legumes.
4. Seek Out Support: Connect with like-minded individuals who share your passion for plant-based nutrition.

Embracing the power of plant-based nutrition will help you unlock the secrets to optimal health, well-being, and vitality. So why wait? Start your journey today and discover the incredible benefits that await you!

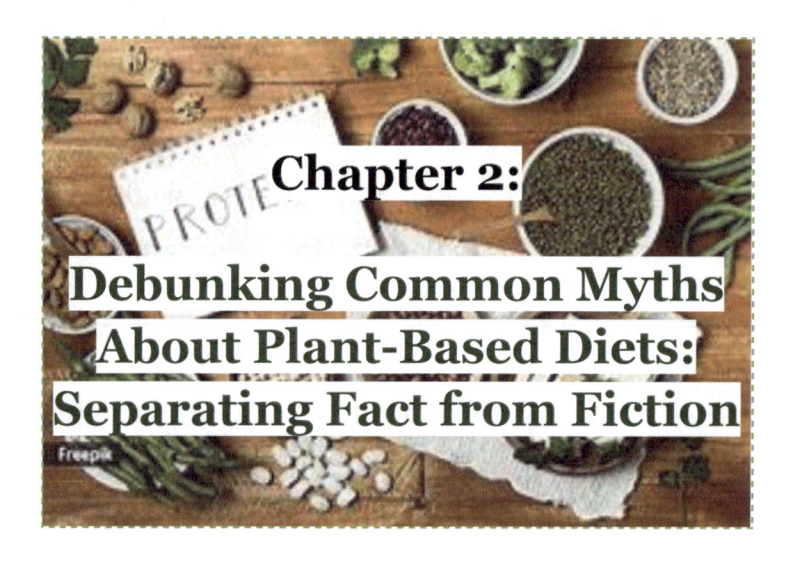

# Chapter 2: Debunking Common Myths About Plant-Based Diets: Separating Fact from Fiction

Are you considering a plant-based diet, but worried about getting enough protein, calcium, or iron? Do you think plant-based diets are boring, tasteless, or expensive? Think again!

As the popularity of plant-based diets continues to grow, so do the misconceptions and myths surrounding this lifestyle choice. It's time to set the record straight and debunk the common myths about plant-based diets.

**Myth #1: Plant-Based Diets Lack Protein**

One of the most enduring myths about plant-based diets is that they're protein-deficient. Nothing could be further from the truth! Plant-based sources of protein are abundant and varied, including:

- Legumes (lentils, chickpeas, black beans)
- Nuts and seeds (almonds, chia seeds, hemp seeds)
- Whole grains (quinoa, brown rice, whole wheat)
- Soy products (tofu, tempeh, edamame)
- Vegetables (broccoli, spinach, kale)

Many plant-based protein sources offer additional nutritional benefits, such as fiber, vitamins, and minerals.

**Myth #2: Plant-Based Diets Are Calcium-Deficient**

Another common myth is that plant-based diets lack calcium, leading to weak bones and osteoporosis. However, plant-based sources of calcium are plentiful, including:

- Dark leafy greens (kale, broccoli, spinach)
- Fortified plant-based milk (soy milk, almond milk, oat milk)
- Tofu and other soy products
- Calcium-set tofu
- Fortified cereals and juices

Many plant-based sources of calcium offer additional nutritional benefits, such as vitamins and minerals.

## Myth #3: Plant-Based Diets Are Iron-Deficient

Iron deficiency is another common concern for those considering a plant-based diet. However, plant-based sources of iron are abundant, including:

- Legumes (lentils, chickpeas, black beans)

- Dark leafy greens (spinach, kale, broccoli)
- Nuts and seeds (pumpkin seeds, sesame seeds, sunflower seeds)
- Whole grains (quinoa, brown rice, whole wheat)
- Fortified cereals and energy bars

Vitamin C can enhance iron absorption, making plant-based sources of iron even more effective.

## Myth #4: Plant-Based Diets Are Boring and Tasteless

Nothing could be further from the truth! Plant-based cuisine is incredibly diverse and flavorful, with a wide range of international cuisines and cooking styles to explore. From spicy Indian curries to hearty Italian pasta dishes, plant-based eating offers endless possibilities for culinary adventure.

## Myth #5: Plant-Based Diets Are Expensive

While some plant-based alternatives to meat and dairy products can be pricey, a well-planned plant-based diet can be incredibly cost-effective. By focusing on whole, minimally processed foods like fruits, vegetables, whole grains, and legumes, you can save money and eat like a king.

## Myth #6: Plant-Based Diets Are Only for Vegans and Vegetarians

Not true! Plant-based diets are for anyone who wants to improve their health, well-being, and environmental sustainability. Whether you're a flexitarian, reducetarian, or just someone who wants to eat more plants, a plant-based diet can be tailored to suit your lifestyle and preferences.

## Myth #7: Plant-Based Diets Are Not Suitable for Athletes or Bodybuilders

Plant-based diets are perfect for athletes and bodybuilders who require high amounts of protein, complex carbohydrates, and healthy fats. Many professional athletes, including tennis champion

Novak Djokovic and NFL player David Carter, thrive on plant-based diets.

## Myth #8: Plant-Based Diets Are Not Suitable for Pregnant or Breastfeeding Women

Plant-based diets can be incredibly beneficial for pregnant and breastfeeding women, providing essential nutrients for fetal development and milk production. However, it's essential to consult with a healthcare professional or registered dietitian to ensure you're getting all the necessary nutrients.

## Myth #9: Plant-Based Diets Are Not Suitable for Children

Plant-based diets can be incredibly beneficial for children, providing essential nutrients for growth and development. A well-planned plant-based diet can help reduce the risk of childhood obesity, allergies, and asthma.

## Myth #10: Plant-Based Diets Are a Fad

Plant-based diets are not a fad; they're a sustainable, long-term solution for optimal health, well-being, and environmental sustainability. With the growing body of scientific evidence supporting the benefits of plant-based eating, it's clear that this lifestyle choice is here to stay.

By debunking these common myths about plant-based diets, we hope to have inspired you to give plant-based eating a try. Whether you're a seasoned vegan or just starting to explore the world of plant-based cuisine, we invite you to join the plant-based revolution and discover the incredible benefits that await you!

# Chapter 3:
## The Benefits of Plant-Based Eating for Weight Loss and Overall Health: Unlocking the Power of Plants

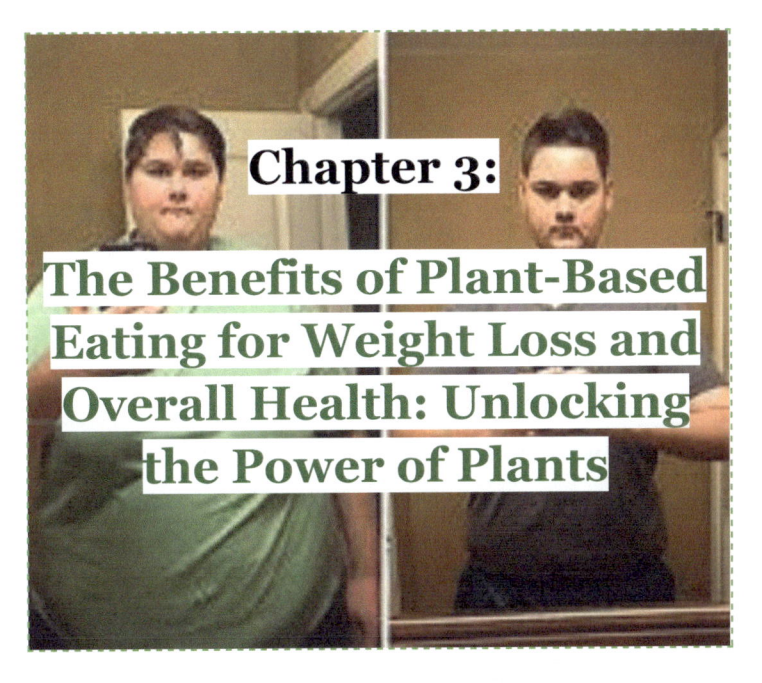

Imagine a world where food is not just sustenance, but a powerful tool for transformation. A world where the nutrients you consume can heal, protect, and energize your body. Welcome to the world of plant-based eating!

Plant-based eating has been shown to have numerous benefits for weight loss and overall health. From boosting your metabolism and energy levels to reducing your risk of chronic diseases and improving your mental clarity and focus, plant-based eating is the key to unlocking your full potential.

**Weight Loss Benefits**

1. Lower Calorie Intake: Plant-based foods tend to be lower in calories and higher in fiber, making it easier to maintain a healthy weight.
2. Increased Satiety: Plant-based foods are rich in fiber, which helps keep you feeling fuller for longer, reducing the likelihood of overeating.
3. Improved Metabolism: Plant-based foods are rich in antioxidants and polyphenols, which help boost your metabolism and support weight loss.
4. Reduced Inflammation*: Plant-based foods are rich in anti-inflammatory compounds, which help reduce inflammation and promote weight loss.

**Overall Health Benefits**
1. Reduced Risk of Chronic Diseases: Plant-based eating has been shown to reduce the risk of chronic diseases like heart disease, type 2 diabetes, and certain types of cancer.
2. Improved Heart Health: Plant-based foods are rich in healthy fats, fiber, and antioxidants, which help support heart health and reduce the risk of cardiovascular disease.
3. Enhanced Mental Clarity and Focus: Plant-based foods are rich in antioxidants, vitamins, and minerals that help support brain health and improve mental clarity and focus.
4. Stronger Immune System: Plant-based foods are rich in antioxidants, vitamins, and minerals that help support immune function and reduce the risk of illness and disease.

**Additional Benefits**
1. Improved Digestion: Plant-based foods are rich in fiber, which helps promote regular bowel movements, prevent constipation, and support healthy gut bacteria.
2. Glowing Skin: Plant-based foods are rich in antioxidants, vitamins, and minerals that help support skin health and reduce the signs of aging.
3. Increased Energy: Plant-based foods are rich in iron, vitamin B12, and other essential nutrients that help support energy production and reduce fatigue.
4. Better Sleep: Plant-based foods are rich in antioxidants, vitamins, and minerals that help support sleep quality and reduce the risk of sleep disorders.

**The Science Behind Plant-Based Eating**

Plant-based eating is not just a diet; it's a lifestyle. It's a choice to fuel your body with the most nutrient-dense, vibrant, and life-affirming foods on the planet. The science behind plant-based eating is clear: a well-planned plant-based diet can provide all the necessary nutrients for optimal health and well-being.

**Getting Started**

1. Start with Small Changes: Begin by incorporating one or two plant-based meals into your diet each day.
2. Explore New Recipes: Try new plant-based recipes and flavors to keep your diet interesting and varied.
3. Seek Out Support: Connect with like-minded individuals who share your passion for plant-based eating.
4. Consult with a Healthcare Professional: Consult with a healthcare professional or registered dietitian to ensure you're getting all the necessary nutrients.

# Part 2: Getting Started with Plant-Based Eating

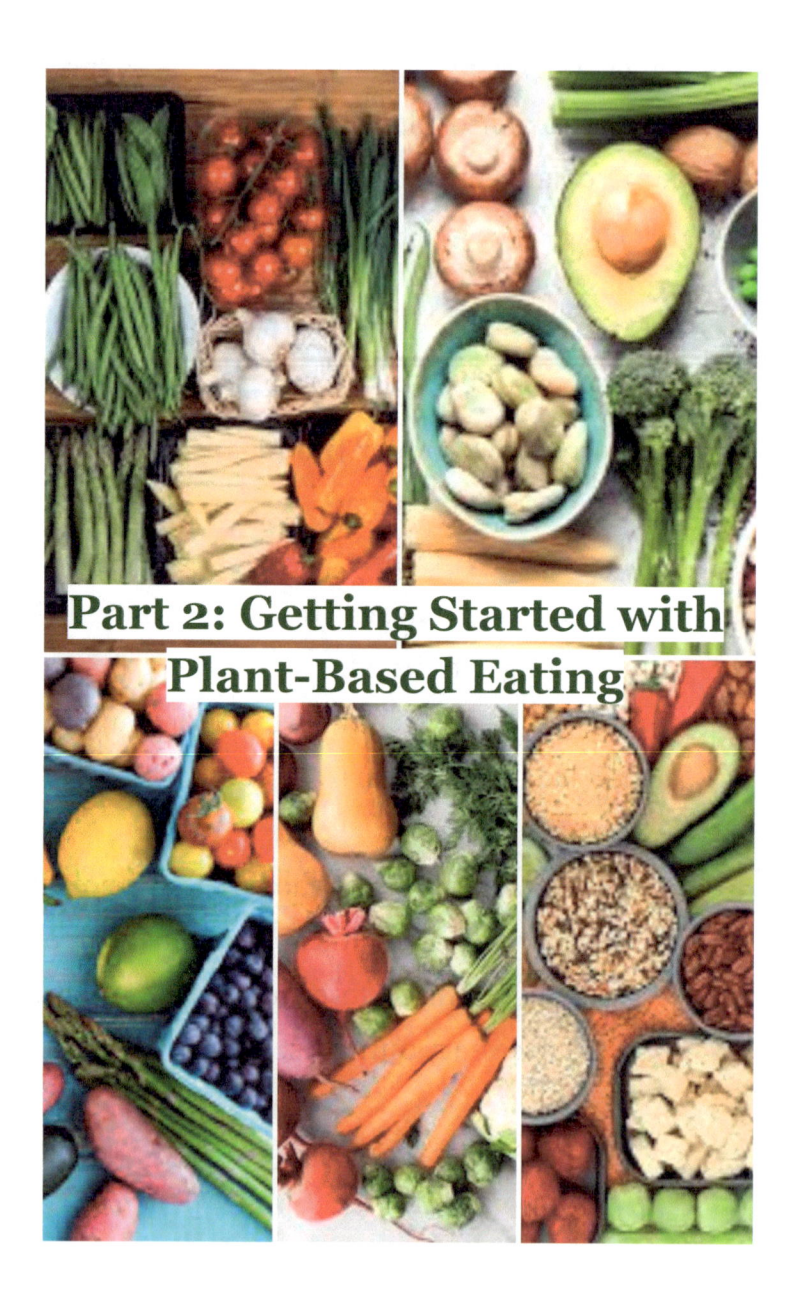

# Chapter 4:

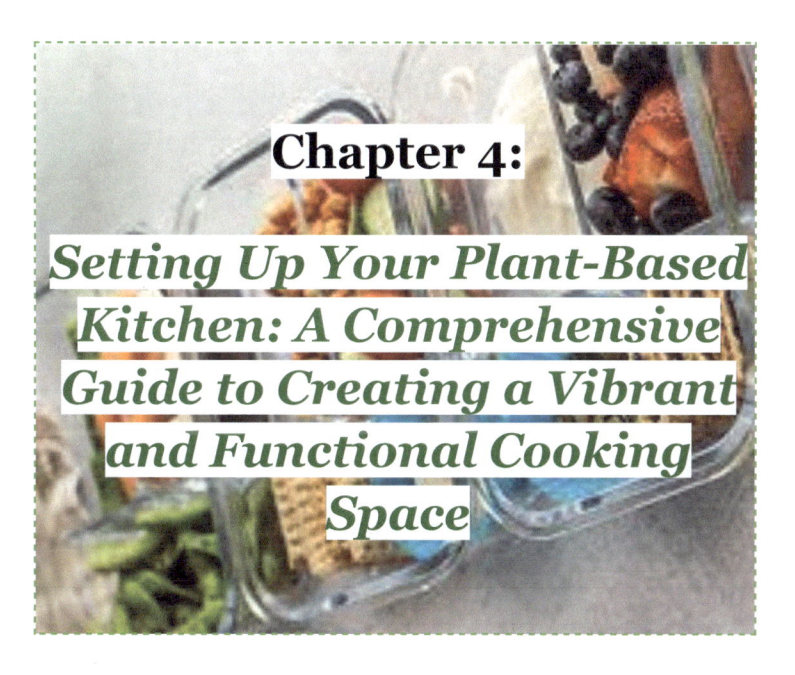

## *Setting Up Your Plant-Based Kitchen: A Comprehensive Guide to Creating a Vibrant and Functional Cooking Space*

Welcome to the heart of your home: the kitchen! As you embark on your plant-based journey, it's essential to create a cooking space that inspires creativity, nourishes your body, and sparks joy. In this comprehensive guide, we'll walk you through setting up your plant-based kitchen, from pantry staples to cooking essentials.

**Pantry Staples: The Foundation of Plant-Based Cooking**

A well-stocked pantry is the backbone of any kitchen. When it comes to plant-based cooking, having the right staples on hand can make all the difference. Here are some essentials to get you started:

1. Grains: Brown rice, quinoa, whole wheat pasta, and oats are all great sources of fiber and nutrients.
2. Canned Goods: Canned beans, tomatoes, and coconut milk are convenient and versatile.
3. Nutritional Yeast: This nutty, cheesy-tasting ingredient is a popular vegan substitute for cheese.
4. Spices and Herbs: Stock up on turmeric, cumin, basil, and oregano to add flavor and depth to your dishes.
5. Plant-Based Milk: Almond milk, soy milk, and oat milk are great dairy alternatives.

## Cooking Essentials: The Tools of the Trade

Now that your pantry is stocked, it's time to focus on the cooking essentials. These tools will help you prepare, cook, and serve delicious plant-based meals with ease:

1. Good Knives: A sharp chef's knife and a paring knife are essential for any kitchen.
2. Cutting Boards: Wooden or bamboo cutting boards are durable and easy to clean.
3. Pots and Pans: Invest in a good stainless steel or cast iron pot and pan for sautéing and cooking.
4. Colander and Strainer: These tools are perfect for draining pasta, rice, and vegetables.
5. Blender and Food Processor: These appliances will help you create smoothies, sauces, and dips with ease.

**Cooking Utensils: The Fun Stuff!**

Now that you have the basics covered, it's time to add some fun and functional cooking utensils to your kitchen:

1. Silicone Spatulas: Heat-resistant and non-stick, these spatulas are perfect for scraping the sides of pots and pans.
2. Wooden Spoons: A set of wooden spoons is essential for stirring, mixing, and tasting.
3. Vegetable Peeler: A good vegetable peeler will make quick work of peeling carrots, zucchini, and other vegetables.
4. Mason Jars: These versatile jars are perfect for storing sauces, soups, and leftovers.
5. Instant Pot or Pressure Cooker: These appliances will help you cook beans, grains, and vegetables quickly and efficiently.

**Kitchen Gadgets: The Nice-to-Haves**

While not essential, these kitchen gadgets can make cooking and preparing plant-based meals a breeze:

1. Spiralizer: Create beautiful zucchini noodles and other vegetable spirals with ease.
2. Dehydrator: Make vegan snacks, such as kale chips and fruit leather.
3. Stand Mixer: A stand mixer will make quick work of mixing, kneading, and whipping.
4. Immersion Blender: Blend soups, sauces, and dips in the pot or container.
5. Rice Cooker: Cook perfect rice, quinoa, and other grains with minimal effort.

**Creating a Functional and Beautiful Kitchen Space**

Now that you have the essentials and nice-to-haves covered, it's time to think about the aesthetics of your kitchen. Here are some tips for creating a functional and beautiful kitchen space:

1. Lighting: Invest in good lighting to illuminate your cooking space.
2. Color Scheme: Choose a color scheme that inspires and makes you happy.

3. Storage: Invest in good storage solutions, such as cabinets, drawers, and shelves.
4. Textiles: Add warmth and texture to your kitchen with textiles, such as towels, aprons, and rugs.
5. Plants: Bring some life and greenery to your kitchen with plants, such as herbs, succulents, or flowers.

Following these tips and guidelines will help you be well on your way to creating a vibrant and functional plant-based kitchen that inspires creativity, nourishes your body, and sparks joy. Happy cooking.

# Chapter 5:

## Stocking Your Pantry with Plant-Based Essentials: A Comprehensive Guide

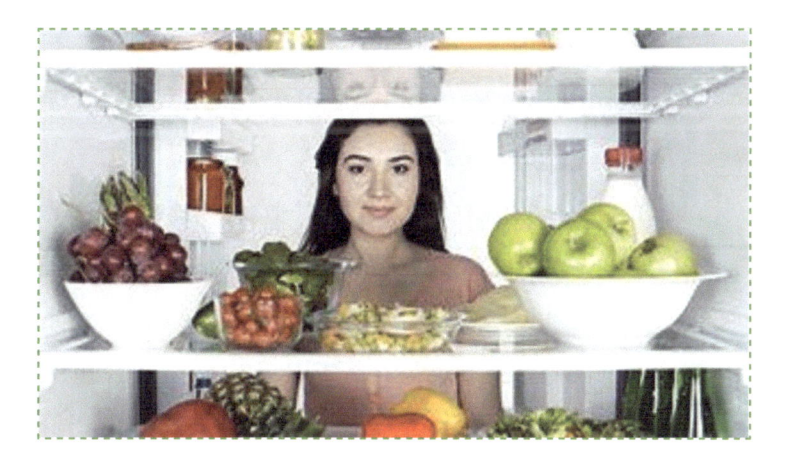

As you embark on your plant-based journey, having a well-stocked pantry is essential for creating delicious, nutritious, and satisfying meals. In this comprehensive guide, we'll explore the must-have plant-based essentials to stock your pantry, making meal prep a breeze.

## The Benefits of a Plant-Based Pantry

Before we dive into the essentials, let's talk about the benefits of a plant-based pantry:

1. Increased food variety: With a well-stocked pantry, you'll have a wide range of ingredients to experiment with, reducing the risk of meal boredom.
2. Improved nutrition: Plant-based ingredients are packed with vitamins, minerals, and antioxidants, fueling your body with the best.
3. Reduced food waste: With a pantry full of staples, you'll be less likely to rely on takeout or processed foods, reducing food waste and saving you money.
4. Simplified meal prep: A well-stocked pantry makes meal prep a breeze, allowing you to whip up healthy meals in no time.

## The Plant-Based Pantry Essentials

Now, let's get to the good stuff! Here are the must-have plant-based essentials to stock your pantry:

1. Grains:
- Brown rice
- Quinoa
- Whole wheat pasta
- Oats

2. Canned Goods:
- Black beans
- Chickpeas
- Canned tomatoes
- Coconut milk

3. Nutritional Powerhouses:
- Nuts (almonds, walnuts, etc.)
- Seeds (chia, flax, etc.)
- Dried fruits (dates, apricots, etc.)

4. Spices and Herbs:
- Turmeric
- Cumin
- Paprika
- Basil
- Oregano

5. Oils and Vinegar:
- Olive oil
- Coconut oil
- Apple cider vinegar
- Balsamic vinegar

6. Plant-Based Milk and Yogurts:
- Almond milk
- Soy milk
- Coconut yogurt
- Cashew yogurt

7. Snacks and Treats:

- Nut butters (peanut butter, almond butter, etc.)
- Dried fruit leather
- Energy balls
- Dark chocolate chips

**Tips for Stocking Your Pantry**

Now that you have the essentials, here are some tips to keep in mind:

1. Buy in bulk: Purchasing items like grains, nuts, and seeds in bulk can save you money and reduce packaging waste.
2. Store properly: Keep your pantry organized and store items in a cool, dry place to maintain freshness.
3. Rotate stock: Regularly rotate your stock to ensure older items are used before they expire.

4. Experiment and have fun: Don't be afraid to try new ingredients and recipes – it's all part of the plant-based journey!

## Conclusion

Stocking your pantry with plant-based essentials is the first step towards creating delicious, nutritious, and satisfying meals. With these must-have ingredients, you'll be well on your way to a healthier, happier you. Remember to buy in bulk, store properly, rotate stock, and most importantly, have fun experimenting with new ingredients and recipes!

# Chapter 6:

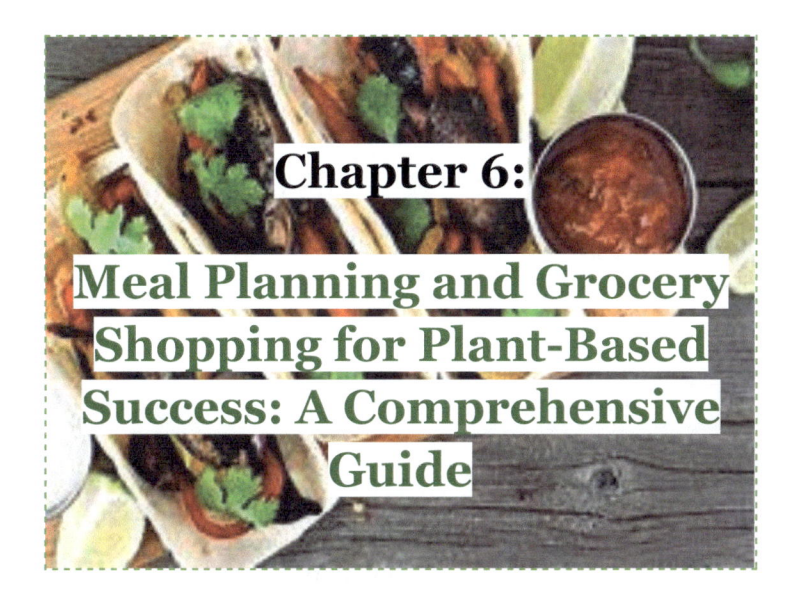

## Meal Planning and Grocery Shopping for Plant-Based Success: A Comprehensive Guide

Congratulations on taking the first step towards a plant-based lifestyle! Meal planning and grocery shopping are essential components of a successful transition. In this guide, we'll walk you through the process of planning delicious, nutritious meals and shopping for the freshest ingredients.

## Why Meal Planning is Crucial

Meal planning is the backbone of a successful plant-based diet. By taking the time to plan your meals, you'll:

1. Save time and money: Avoid last-minute takeout or dining out by having a plan in place.
2. Reduce food waste: Plan meals around ingredients you already have, reducing waste and saving you money.
3. Ensure nutritional balance: Plan meals that include a variety of nutrient-dense foods to ensure you're getting all the necessary vitamins and minerals.
4. Stay on track: A meal plan helps you stay committed to your plant-based goals, even on busy days.

## How to Create a Meal Plan

Creating a meal plan is easier than you think! Follow these simple steps:

1. Determine your dietary needs: Consider your lifestyle, dietary restrictions, and nutritional goals.
2. Choose a meal planning template: Find a template online or create your own using a spreadsheet or calendar.
3. Plan your meals: Start by planning breakfast, lunch, and dinner for each day of the week. Include snacks and desserts if needed.
4. Make a grocery list: Write down the ingredients needed for each meal and snack.
5. Review and adjust: Review your meal plan and make adjustments as needed.

## Grocery Shopping for Plant-Based Success

Grocery shopping can be overwhelming, especially when transitioning to a plant-based diet. Here are some tips to help you shop like a pro:

1. Shop the perimeter of the store: Focus on whole, unprocessed foods like fruits, vegetables, whole grains, and legumes.
2. Read labels: Be mindful of ingredients and choose products with minimal processing and no animal-derived ingredients.
3. Buy in bulk: Purchasing items like grains, nuts, and seeds in bulk can save you money and reduce packaging waste.
4. Shop seasonal: Choose produce that's in season to ensure freshness and affordability.
5. Don't forget the staples: Make sure to stock up on plant-based staples like canned beans, nutritional yeast, and plant-based milk.

## Tips for Shopping on a Budget

Eating plant-based doesn't have to break the bank! Here are some tips for shopping on a budget:

1. Plan your meals around sales: Check the weekly ads for your local grocery stores and plan your meals around the items on sale.
2. Use coupons and discount codes: Take advantage of digital coupons, discount codes, and cashback apps to save even more.
3. Shop at local farmer's markets: Many farmers markets offer affordable, fresh produce and a chance to connect with local farmers.
4. Buy in bulk with friends: Split bulk purchases with friends or family members to reduce costs and waste.

## Conclusion

Meal planning and grocery shopping are essential components of a successful plant-based lifestyle. By taking the time to plan your meals and shop for whole, unprocessed foods, you'll be well on your way to achieving your health and wellness goals. Remember to stay flexible, have fun, and enjoy the journey!

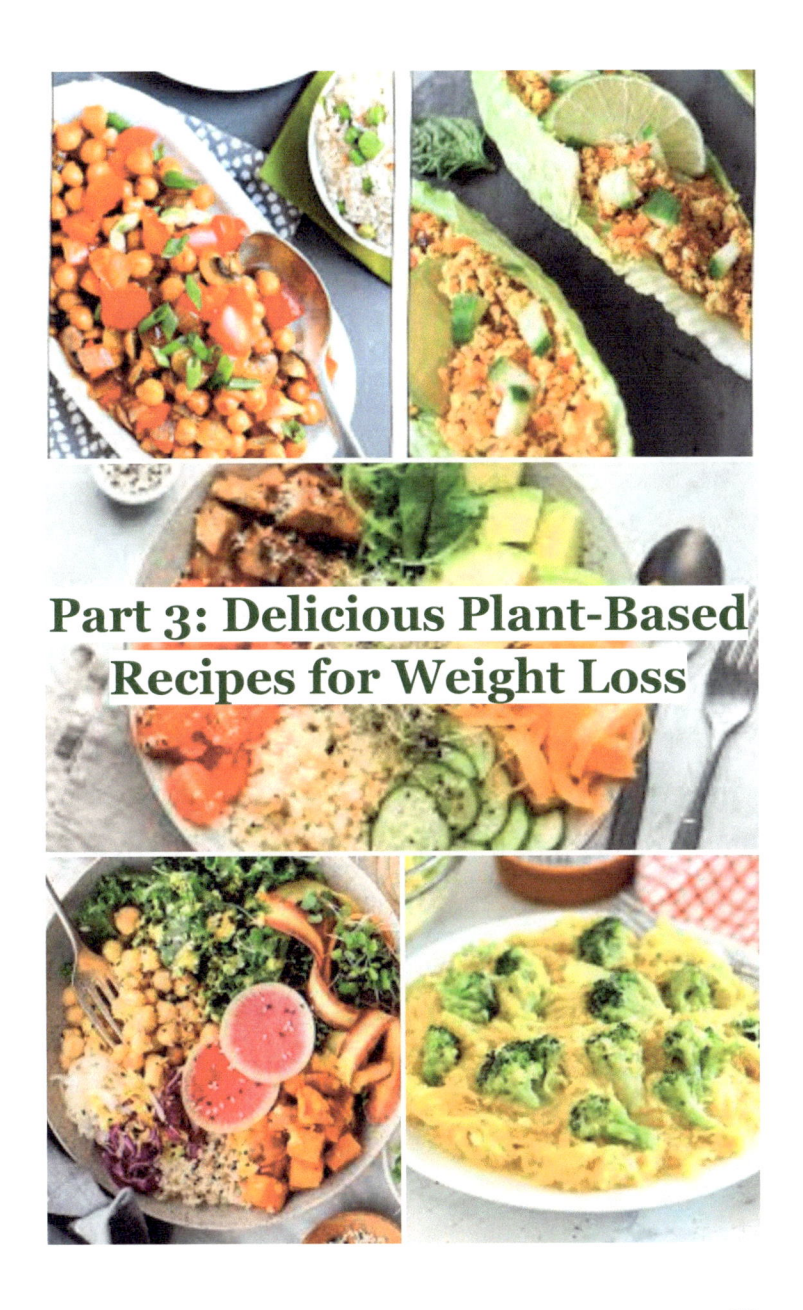

# Part 3: Delicious Plant-Based Recipes for Weight Loss

# Chapter 7:

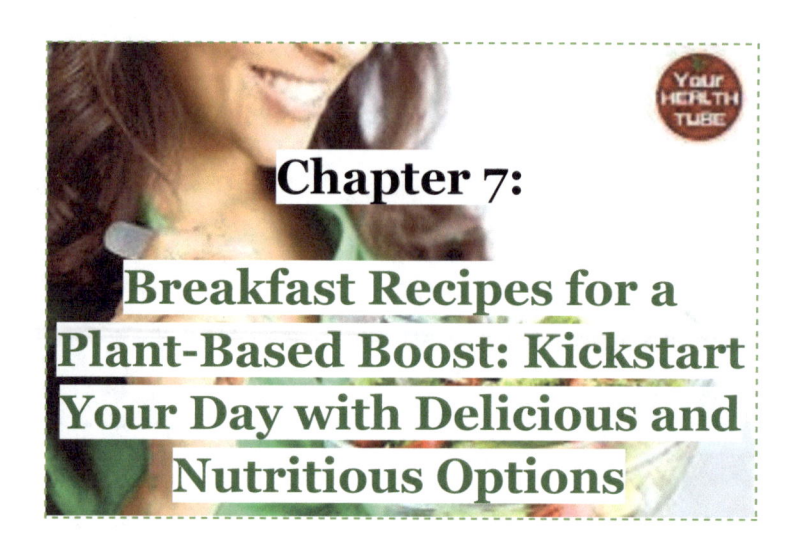

## Breakfast Recipes for a Plant-Based Boost: Kickstart Your Day with Delicious and Nutritious Options

Breakfast-the most important meal of the day! A nutritious breakfast can boost your energy, jumpstart your metabolism, and set you up for a day of vitality and focus. As a plant-based enthusiast, you're in luck! We've got a treasure trove of mouth-watering, nutrient-dense breakfast recipes to kickstart your day.

**Why Plant-Based Breakfasts Rock**

Before we dive into the recipes, let's explore why plant-based breakfasts are an excellent choice:

1. High fiber content: Plant-based breakfasts are packed with fiber-rich foods like fruits, whole grains, and legumes, which can help lower cholesterol and regulate blood sugar.
2. Antioxidant-rich: Plant-based breakfasts are bursting with antioxidants from fruits, vegetables, and whole grains, which can help protect against chronic diseases like cancer and heart disease.
3. Inflammation-fighting: Many plant-based breakfast ingredients, such as turmeric and ginger, have potent anti-inflammatory properties that can help reduce inflammation and promote overall well-being.
4. Weight management: Plant-based breakfasts tend to be lower in calories and higher in fiber, making them an excellent choice for those looking to manage their weight.

## 15 Plant-Based Breakfast Recipes to Boost Your Day

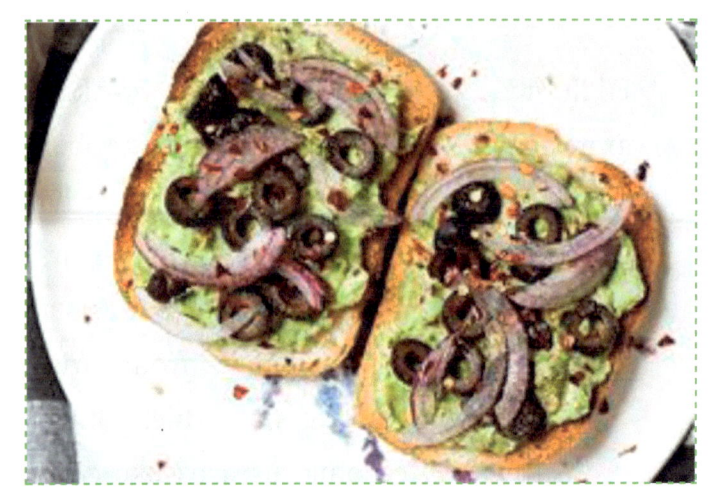

Now, let's get to the fun part! Here are 15 delicious and nutritious plant-based breakfast recipes to kickstart your day:

1. Avocado Toast: Toast whole grain bread, mash avocado, and sprinkle with salt, pepper, and a squeeze of lemon juice.
2. Chia Seed Pudding: Mix chia seeds with almond milk, honey, and vanilla extract, then refrigerate overnight and top with fresh fruit.

3. Quinoa Breakfast Bowl: Cook quinoa and mix with diced veggies, nuts, and seeds, then top with a citrus-tahini dressing.
4. Green Smoothie: Blend your favorite greens, fruits, and plant-based milk for a nutrient-packed breakfast on the go.
5. Whole Grain Waffles: Make whole grain waffles and top with fresh fruit, nut butter, or a drizzle of maple syrup.
6. Lentil Breakfast Curry: Cook lentils with onions, ginger, and spices, then serve with whole grain toast or over rice.
7. Roasted Veggie Omelette: Whisk together tofu, nutritional yeast, and spices, then fill with roasted veggies and cook into an omelet.
8. Cinnamon Apple Oatmeal: Cook oatmeal with cinnamon, apple, and a hint of nutmeg, then top with fresh fruit and a drizzle of maple syrup.
9. Chickpea Scramble: Scramble chickpeas with turmeric, nutritional yeast, and spices, then

serve with whole grain toast or wrapped in a whole grain tortilla.

10. Banana Nice Cream: Freeze bananas and blend into a creamy "ice cream," then top with fresh fruit, nuts, or shredded coconut.
11. Spinach and Mushroom Quiche: Mix cooked spinach, mushrooms, and tofu with whole grain crust and bake into a savory quiche.
12. Peanut Butter Banana Toast: Toast whole grain bread, spread with peanut butter, and top with sliced banana.
13. Whole Grain Pancakes: Make whole grain pancakes and top with fresh fruit, nut butter, or a drizzle of maple syrup.
14. Kale and Lemon Smoothie: Blend kale, lemon juice, and plant-based milk for a refreshing and nutritious breakfast smoothie.
15. Breakfast Burrito: Scramble tofu with spices, then wrap in a whole grain tortilla with roasted veggies, avocado, and salsa.

**Tips for Meal Planning and Grocery Shopping**

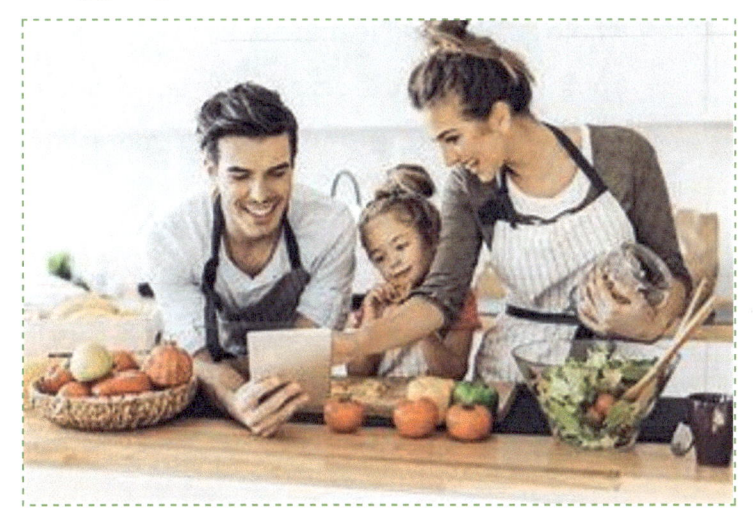

To make meal planning and grocery shopping a breeze, remember these tips:
1. Plan your meals around seasonal produce_: Check your local farmer's market or grocery store to see what's in season, then plan your meals accordingly.
2. Make a grocery list and stick to it: Avoid impulse buys by making a list and sticking to it.

3. Shop the perimeter of the store: Focus on whole, unprocessed foods like fruits, veggies, whole grains, and legumes.
4. Cook in bulk and freeze: Cook large batches of breakfast recipes and freeze them for later, saving you time and money.

**Final Thoughts**

Breakfast is the perfect meal to kickstart your day with a plant-based boost! With these 15 delicious and nutritious breakfast recipes, you'll be well on your way to a vibrant and energized morning. Remember to plan your meals, shop smart, and cook in bulk to make the most of your plant-based breakfast routine. Happy cooking!

# Chapter 8:

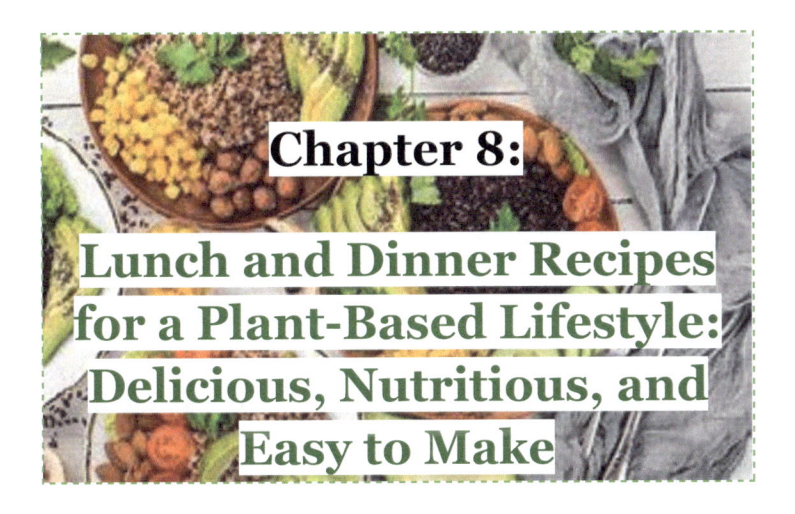

## Lunch and Dinner Recipes for a Plant-Based Lifestyle: Delicious, Nutritious, and Easy to Make

As you continue on your plant-based journey, you're probably eager to explore more delicious and nutritious recipes to fuel your body. In this comprehensive guide, we'll dive into the world of lunch and dinner recipes, showcasing a variety of mouth-watering, easy-to-make dishes that are perfect for a plant-based lifestyle.

## Why Plant-Based Lunches and Dinners Matter

Before we dive into the recipes, let's explore why plant-based lunches and dinners are essential for a healthy and balanced lifestyle:

1. Boosts energy and productivity: Plant-based lunches and dinners provide sustained energy and support mental clarity, helping you power through your day.
2. Supports weight management: Plant-based meals tend to be lower in calories and higher in fiber, making it easier to maintain a healthy weight.
3. Reduces chronic disease risk: A plant-based diet has been shown to reduce the risk of chronic diseases like heart disease, type 2 diabetes, and certain types of cancer.
4. Promotes gut health: Plant-based meals are rich in fiber, which supports the growth of

beneficial gut bacteria and promotes a healthy gut microbiome.

**Lunch Recipes for a Plant-Based Lifestyle**

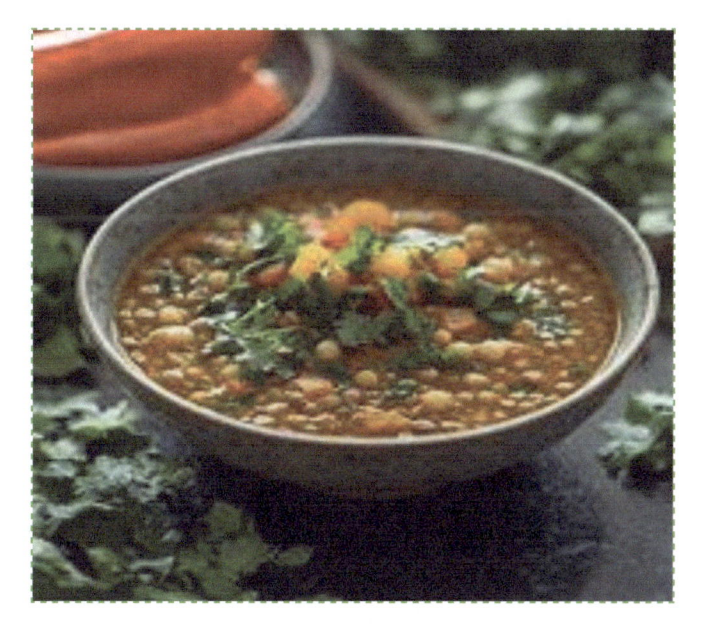

Here are 15 delicious and nutritious plant-based lunch recipes to inspire your meal prep:

1. Veggie Wraps: Fill whole grain wraps with roasted veggies, hummus, and mixed greens.

2. Quinoa Salad Bowls: Mix cooked quinoa with roasted veggies, chickpeas, and a citrus-tahini dressing.
3. Lentil Soup: Cook lentils with veggies and spices, then serve with whole grain bread or crackers.
4. Grilled Veggie Sandwiches: Grill sliced veggies and layer on whole grain bread with hummus and avocado.
5. Chickpea Salad: Mix cooked chickpeas with diced veggies, lemon juice, and olive oil.
6. Roasted Veggie Bowls: Roast a variety of veggies and serve over quinoa or brown rice.
7. Falafel Wrap: Fill a whole-grain wrap with falafel, hummus, and mixed greens.
8. Spinach and Artichoke Wrap: Fill a whole-grain wrap with spinach, artichoke hearts, and hummus.
9. Veggie and Bean Chili: Cook a hearty chili with a variety of veggies and beans.

10. Quinoa and Black Bean Bowl: Mix cooked quinoa and black beans with roasted veggies and a drizzle of tahini sauce.
11. Grilled Portobello Mushroom Burgers: Marinate and grill portobello mushrooms, then serve on a whole grain bun with your favorite toppings.
12. Lentil and Veggie Curry: Cook lentils and veggies in a flavorful curry sauce, served over brown rice or with whole grain naan.
13. Chickpea and Avocado Salad: Mix cooked chickpeas with diced avocado, lemon juice, and olive oil.
14. Roasted Veggie and Quinoa Bowl: Roast a variety of veggies and serve over quinoa with a drizzle of tahini sauce.
15. Veggie and Bean Tacos: Cook a variety of veggies and beans, then serve in whole grain tacos with your favorite toppings.

**Dinner Recipes for a Plant-Based Lifestyle**

**Here are 15 delicious and nutritious plant-based dinner recipes to inspire your meal prep:**

1. Veggie Stir-Fry: Stir-fry a variety of veggies with tofu and brown rice.
2. Lentil and Mushroom Bolognese: Cook lentils and mushrooms in a rich tomato sauce, served over whole grain pasta.
3. Roasted Veggie Bowl: Roast a variety of veggies and serve over quinoa or brown rice.
4. Chickpea and Spinach Curry: Cook chickpeas and spinach in a flavorful curry sauce, served over brown rice or with whole grain naan.
5. Grilled Portobello Mushroom Steaks: Marinate and grill portobello mushrooms, then serve with roasted veggies and quinoa.
6. Veggie and Bean Chili: Cook a hearty chili with a variety of veggies and beans.

7. Quinoa and Black Bean Bowl: Mix cooked quinoa and black beans with roasted veggies and a drizzle of tahini sauce.
8. Lentil and Veggie Shepherd's Pie: Cook lentils and veggies in a rich tomato sauce, top with mashed potatoes, and bake until golden brown.
9. Chickpea and Avocado Salad: Mix cooked chickpeas with diced avocado, lemon juice, and olive oil.
10. Roasted Veggie and Quinoa Bowl: Roast a variety of veggies and serve over quinoa with a drizzle of tahini sauce.
11. Veggie and Bean Tacos: Cook a variety of veggies and beans, then serve in whole grain tacos with your favorite toppings.
12. Stuffed Bell Peppers: Fill bell peppers with a mixture of cooked rice, black beans, and veggies, then bake until tender.
13. Lentil and Mushroom Bourguignon: Cook lentils and mushrooms in a rich, flavorful

broth, served over whole grain bread or with whole grain noodles.

14. Chickpea and Spinach Stew: Cook chickpeas and spinach in a hearty, comforting stew, served with whole grain bread or over brown rice.

15. Veggie and Bean Quesadillas: Fill whole grain tortillas with a mixture of cooked veggies and beans, then cook until crispy and serve with your favorite toppings.

## Tips for Meal Planning and Grocery Shopping

To make meal planning and grocery shopping a breeze, remember these tips:

1. Plan your meals around seasonal produce: Check your local farmer's market or grocery

store to see what's in season, then plan your meals accordingly.
2. Make a grocery list and stick to it: Avoid impulse buys by making a list and sticking to it.
3. Shop the perimeter of the store: Focus on whole, unprocessed foods like fruits, veggies, whole grains, and legumes.
4. Cook in bulk and freeze: Cook large batches of meals and freeze them for later, saving you time and money.

**Final Thought**

Lunch and dinner are essential meals for a plant-based lifestyle, providing sustained energy and supporting overall health and well-being. With these 30 delicious and nutritious recipes, you'll be well on your way to creating a balanced and satisfying plant-based diet. Remember to plan your meals, shop smart, and cook in bulk to make the most of your plant-based lifestyle. Happy cooking!

# Chapter 9:

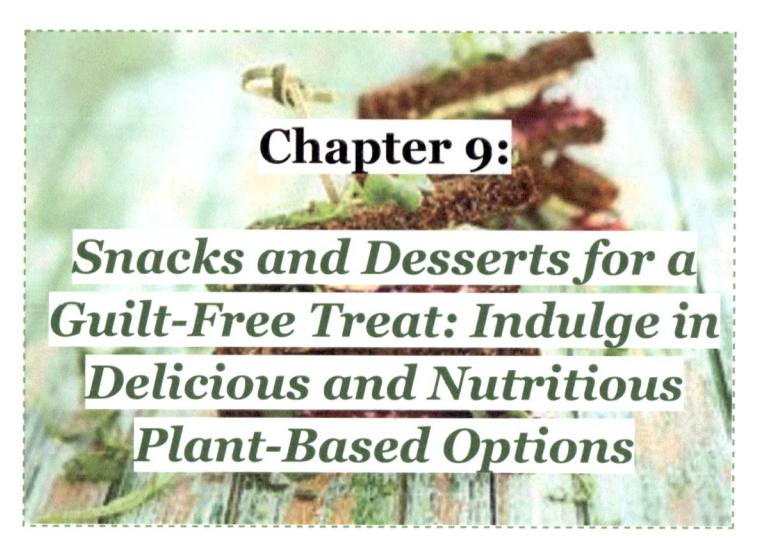

# Snacks and Desserts for a Guilt-Free Treat: Indulge in Delicious and Nutritious Plant-Based Options

Who says you can't have your cake and eat it too? With plant-based snacks and desserts, you can indulge in delicious and nutritious treats that are not only guilt-free but also beneficial for your overall health and well-being.

**Why Plant-Based Snacks and Desserts Matter**

Before we dive into the recipes, let's explore why plant-based snacks and desserts are essential for a healthy and balanced lifestyle:

1. Satisfies cravings: Plant-based snacks and desserts can satisfy your cravings for sweet or savory treats without compromising your dietary goals.
2. Boosts energy: Many plant-based snacks and desserts are rich in nutrients, fiber, and antioxidants, which can help boost your energy levels and support overall health.
3. Supports weight management: Plant-based snacks and desserts tend to be lower in calories and higher in fiber, making them an excellent choice for those looking to manage their weight.
4. Promotes healthy digestion: Plant-based snacks and desserts are often rich in fiber, which can help promote healthy digestion, prevent constipation, and support the growth of beneficial gut bacteria.

## Plant-Based Snack Recipes

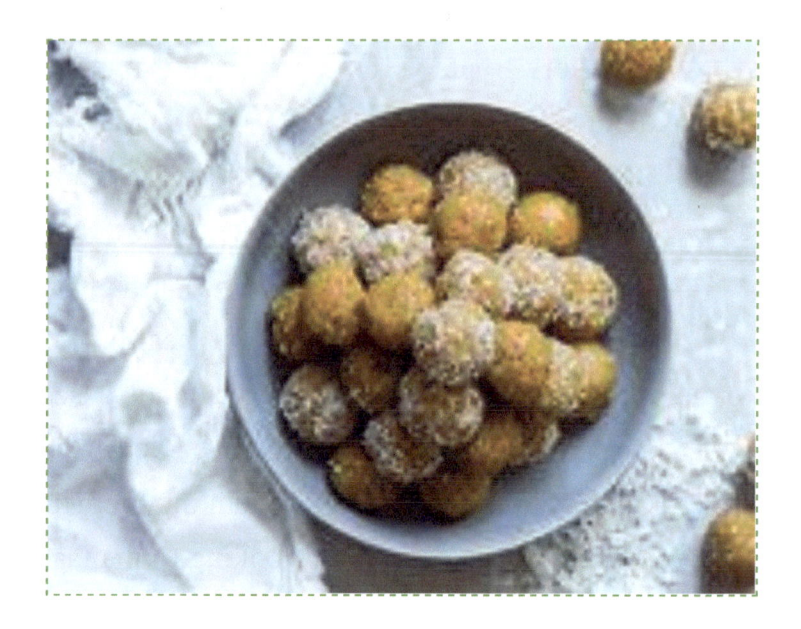

Here are 15 delicious and nutritious plant-based snack recipes to satisfy your cravings:

1. Spicy Roasted Chickpeas: Roast chickpeas with spices and herbs for a crunchy and addictive snack.

2. Fresh Fruit Skewers: Skewer fresh fruit like grapes, strawberries, and pineapple for a healthy and colorful snack.
3. Energy Balls: Mix rolled oats, nuts, and dried fruit to create bite-sized energy balls that are perfect for on-the-go snacking.
4. Hummus and Veggie Sticks: Dip raw or roasted veggie sticks in a creamy and protein-rich hummus.
5. Trail Mix: Mix nuts, seeds, and dried fruit for a healthy and convenient snack that's perfect for hiking or traveling.
6. Quinoa Bites: Mix cooked quinoa with nuts, seeds, and dried fruit to create crunchy and nutritious bite-sized snacks.
7. Smoothie Bowls: Blend your favorite fruits and toppings, then top with granola, nuts, and seeds for a nutritious and filling snack.
8. Roasted Veggie Chips: Roast sliced veggies like sweet potatoes or beets for a crispy and addictive snack.

9. Edamame and Mango Salad: Mix cooked edamame with diced mango, red onion, and a squeeze of lime juice for a refreshing and protein-rich snack.
10. Chia Seed Pudding: Mix chia seeds with plant-based milk and let it sit overnight for a healthy and filling snack.
11. Cinnamon Apple Slices: Dip sliced apples in a mixture of cinnamon and nutmeg for a healthy and delicious snack.
12. Lentil or Black Bean Dip: Mix cooked lentils or black beans with spices and herbs for a protein-rich and delicious dip.
13. Grilled Veggie Skewers: Skewer marinated veggies like bell peppers, zucchini, and onions, then grill until tender.
14. Quinoa and Black Bean Salad: Mix cooked quinoa and black beans with diced veggies and a squeeze of lime juice for a healthy and filling snack.

15. No-Bake Energy Bars: Mix rolled oats, nuts, and dried fruit to create no-bake energy bars that are perfect for on-the-go snacking.

**Plant-Based Dessert Recipes**

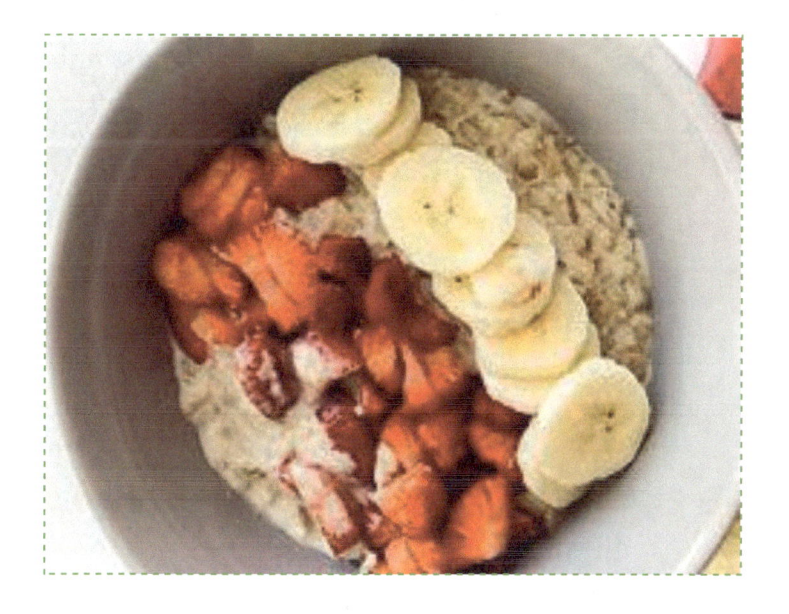

Here are 15 delicious and nutritious plant-based dessert recipes to satisfy your sweet tooth:

1. Chocolate Chia Seed Pudding: Mix chia seeds with plant-based milk, cocoa powder, and maple syrup for a rich and decadent dessert.
2. Berry Sorbet: Blend frozen berries with a squeeze of lemon juice and a drizzle of maple syrup for a light and refreshing dessert.
3. No-Bake Energy Bites: Mix rolled oats, nuts, and dried fruit to create bite-sized energy balls that are perfect for a sweet treat.
4. Coconut Lime Tarts: Mix coconut cream with lime juice and maple syrup, then fill pre-made tart crusts for a creamy and tangy dessert.
5. Banana Nice Cream: Freeze bananas and blend into a creamy "ice cream," then top with your favorite toppings.
6. Apple Crisp: Mix sliced apples with oats, nuts, and spices, then bake until tender and top with a crunchy oat topping.
7. Chocolate Avocado Mousse: Mix ripe avocados with cocoa powder, maple syrup,

and coconut cream for a rich and creamy dessert.

8. Pecan Pie Bars: Mix pecans with maple syrup, coconut sugar, and coconut oil, then press into a pre-made crust for a delicious and nutritious dessert.
9. Raspberry Galette: Mix fresh raspberries with coconut sugar and lemon juice, then fill a pre-made crust and bake until golden brown.

10. Chocolate Chip Cookie Dough Balls: Mix rolled oats, nut butter, and chocolate chips to create bite-sized cookie dough balls that are perfect for a sweet treat.

11. Pistachio and Rosewater Macarons: Mix ground pistachios with rosewater and coconut sugar, then fill pre-made macaron shells for a delicate and exotic dessert.

12. No-Bake Peanut Butter Bars: Mix rolled oats, peanut butter, and coconut sugar, then press into a pre-made crust for a creamy and indulgent dessert.

13. Cinnamon Apple Crumble: Mix sliced apples with cinnamon, nutmeg, and coconut sugar, then top with a crunchy oat topping and bake until golden brown.

14. Chocolate Banana Nice Cream Sandwiches: Freeze bananas and blend them into a creamy "ice cream," then sandwich between two cookies or wafers for a decadent dessert.

15. Lemon Bars with a Shortbread Crust: Mix a shortbread crust with a lemon filling made from coconut cream, lemon juice, and maple syrup, then bake until golden brown.

## Tips for Making Delicious Plant-Based Snacks and Desserts

To make delicious plant-based snacks and desserts, remember these tips:

1. Experiment with new ingredients: Try new fruits, nuts, and spices to create unique and delicious flavor combinations.
2. Use natural sweeteners: Choose natural sweeteners like maple syrup, coconut sugar, and dates instead of refined sugars.
3. Don't be afraid of fat: Use healthy fats like coconut oil, nut butter, and avocado to add creaminess and flavor to your snacks and desserts.
4. Keep it simple: Don't be intimidated by complex recipes – simple snacks and desserts can be just as delicious and satisfying.

**Conclusion**

Plant-based snacks and desserts are not only delicious, but they're also nutritious and beneficial for your overall health and well-being. With these 30 recipes, you'll be well on your way to creating a balanced and satisfying plant-based diet that's free from guilt and full of flavor. Happy snacking and indulging!

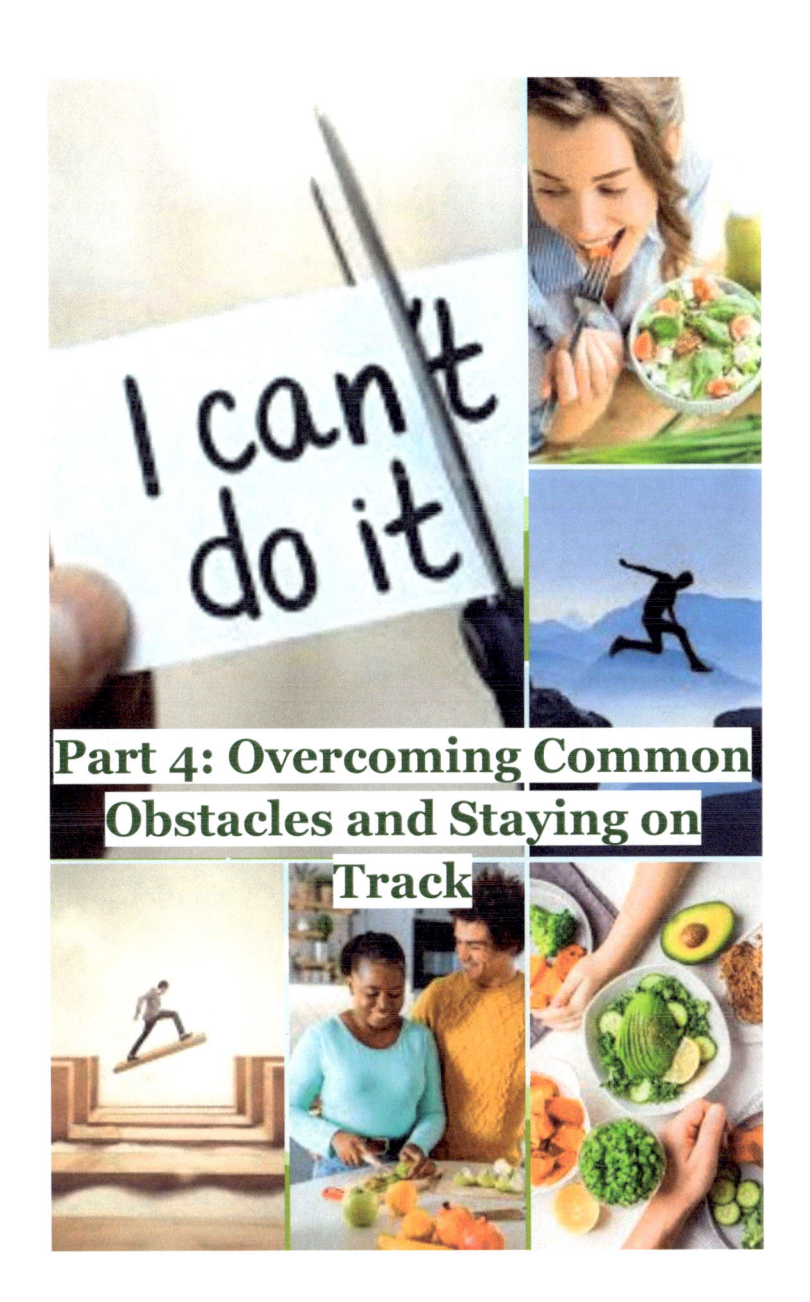

# Part 4: Overcoming Common Obstacles and Staying on Track

# Chapter 10:

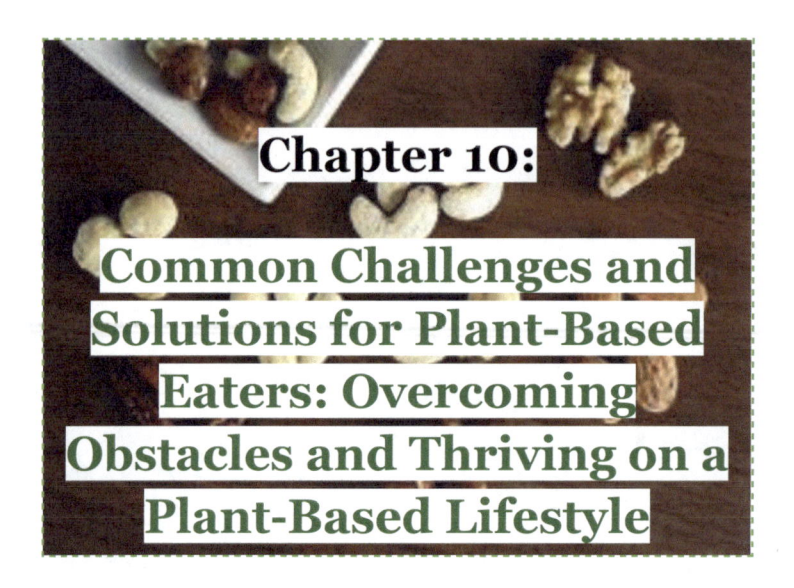

## Common Challenges and Solutions for Plant-Based Eaters: Overcoming Obstacles and Thriving on a Plant-Based Lifestyle

As you embark on your plant-based journey, you may encounter some challenges that can make it difficult to stick to your new lifestyle. Don't worry, you're not alone! Many plant-based eaters face similar obstacles, and with the right solutions, you can overcome them and thrive on a plant-based diet.

**Challenge 1: Protein Deficiency**

One of the most common concerns about plant-based diets is protein deficiency. Many people believe that plant-based sources of protein are inadequate, but this couldn't be further from the truth.

**Solutions:**

1. Eat a variety of protein-rich foods: Include a variety of protein-rich foods like legumes, beans, lentils, tofu, tempeh, and seitan in your diet.
2. Combine protein sources: Combine different protein sources like whole grains and legumes to create complete proteins.
3. Consult with a registered dietitian or nutritionist: A registered dietitian or nutritionist can help you create a personalized meal plan that meets your protein needs.

## Challenge 2: Vitamin B12 Deficiency

Vitamin B12 is an essential nutrient that plays a critical role in the production of red blood cells and the maintenance of the nervous system. Since vitamin B12 is primarily found in animal products, plant-based eaters may be at risk of deficiency.

**Solutions:**

1. Take a vitamin B12 supplement: Consider taking a vitamin B12 supplement to ensure you're getting enough of this essential nutrient.
2. Eat fortified foods: Many plant-based milk and cereals are fortified with vitamin B12, so be sure to include these in your diet.
3. Consult with a registered dietitian or nutritionist: A registered dietitian or nutritionist can help you create a personalized meal plan that meets your vitamin B12 needs.

## Challenge 3: Social Challenges

One of the biggest challenges plant-based eaters face is social pressure. Whether it's dining out with friends or attending family gatherings, it can be difficult to stick to your plant-based diet in social situations.

## Solutions:

1. Communicate with your friends and family: Let your friends and family know about your plant-based diet and ask for their support.
2. Offer to bring a dish: When attending social gatherings, offer to bring a plant-based dish to share with others.
3. Find plant-based-friendly restaurants: Research plant-based-friendly restaurants in your area and suggest them when dining out with friends.

## Challenge 4: Cravings and Temptation

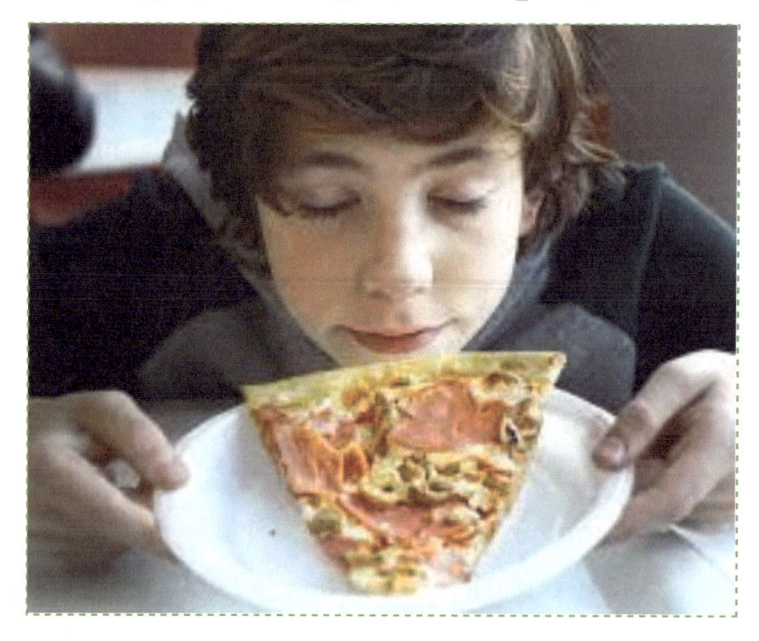

Let's face it – cravings and temptation can be a real challenge for plant-based eaters. Whether it's a craving for cheese or a temptation to try non-plant-based food, it can be difficult to stick to your diet.

**Solutions:**

1. Find healthy alternatives: Find healthy plant-based alternatives to your favorite non-plant-based foods.
2. Plan: Plan your meals and snacks to avoid temptation.
3. Seek support: Share your struggles with a friend or family member and ask for their support.

**Challenge 5: Nutrient Deficiencies**

Plant-based eaters may be at risk of nutrient deficiencies if they don't plan their diet carefully. Common nutrient deficiencies include iron, zinc, and omega-3 fatty acids.

**Solutions:**
1. Eat a variety of nutrient-dense foods: Include a variety of nutrient-dense foods like whole grains, legumes, and leafy greens in your diet.

2. Consult with a registered dietitian or nutritionist: A registered dietitian or nutritionist can help you create a personalized meal plan that meets your nutrient needs.
3. Take supplements if necessary: If you're unable to get enough of a particular nutrient from your diet, consider taking a supplement.

**Conclusion**

While challenges may arise on your plant-based journey, they're not insurmountable. By being aware of the common challenges and solutions, you can overcome obstacles and thrive on a plant-based lifestyle. Remember to stay positive, seek support, and be patient with yourself as you navigate the world of plant-based eating. Happy eating!

# Chapter 11:

## Staying Motivated and Accountable on Your Plant-Based Journey: A Comprehensive Guide to Achieving Long-Term Success

Congratulations on taking the first step towards a healthier, more compassionate lifestyle! As you embark on your plant-based journey, it's essential to stay motivated and accountable to ensure long-term success. In this comprehensive guide, we'll explore the tips, strategies, and inspiration you need to stay on track and achieve your plant-based goals.

## The Importance of Motivation and Accountability

Staying motivated and accountable is crucial to achieving success on your plant-based journey. Here are just a few reasons why:

1. Increased chances of success: When you're motivated and accountable, you're more likely to stick to your plant-based diet and achieve your health and wellness goals.
2. Improved mental and physical health: A plant-based diet has been shown to have numerous physical and mental health benefits, including reduced inflammation, improved heart health, and increased energy levels.
3. Increased self-confidence: When you're able to stick to your plant-based diet and achieve your goals, you'll feel more confident and empowered to take control of your health and wellness.

4. Better habits and routines: Staying motivated and accountable helps you develop better habits and routines, including meal planning, grocery shopping, and cooking.

**Tips for Staying Motivated**

Here are some tips to help you stay motivated on your plant-based journey:

1. Set clear goals: Define your why and set specific, measurable, achievable, relevant, and time-bound (SMART) goals for yourself.
2. Track your progress: Keep a food diary or use a mobile app to track your progress and stay accountable.
3. Celebrate milestones: Celebrate your milestones, no matter how small they may seem, to stay motivated and encouraged.
4. Find a plant-based community: Connect with other plant-based individuals through online

communities, social media groups, or local meetups.
5. Reward yourself: Reward yourself for reaching milestones and staying on track with non-food-related rewards, such as a new book or a relaxing bath.

**Tips for Staying Accountable**

Here are some tips to help you stay accountable on your plant-based journey:

1. Get a plant-based buddy: Find a friend or family member who shares your plant-based goals and values, and support each other on your journey.
2. Hire a health coach or nutritionist: Work with a health coach or nutritionist who can provide personalized guidance and support.
3. Join a plant-based challenge or program: Join a plant-based challenge or program that provides structure and accountability.

4. Share your journey with friends and family: Share your plant-based journey with friends and family, and ask for their support and encouragement.

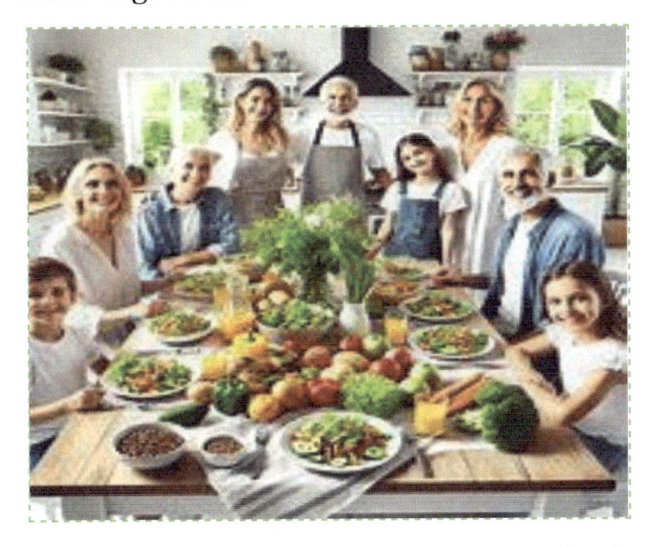

5. Be kind to yourself: Remember that setbacks are a normal part of the journey, and be kind to yourself when you make mistakes.

## Strategies for Overcoming Common Challenges

Here are some strategies for overcoming common challenges on your plant-based journey:

1. Meal planning and prep: Plan your meals and prep in advance to avoid last-minute temptations.
2. Eating out and social situations: Research plant-based-friendly restaurants and social situations, and don't be afraid to ask for modifications or substitutions.
3. Cravings and temptations: Find healthy alternatives to your favorite comfort foods, and stay hydrated and satisfied with nutrient-dense snacks.
4. Lack of motivation and accountability: Find a plant-based community or buddy, and track your progress to stay motivated and accountable.

5. Nutrient deficiencies and health concerns: Consult with a registered dietitian or nutritionist to ensure you're getting all the necessary nutrients and address any health concerns.

**Inspiration and Motivation**

Here are some inspiring stories and motivational quotes to keep you on track:

1. Success stories: Read inspiring stories of people who have achieved success on their plant-based journey.
2. Motivational quotes: Read motivational quotes from plant-based leaders and experts.
3. Plant-based influencers and bloggers: Follow plant-based influencers and bloggers who share inspiring stories, recipes, and tips.
4. Documentaries and films: Watch documentaries and films that showcase the benefits of a plant-based lifestyle.

5. Plant-based events and conferences: Attend plant-based events and conferences to connect with like-minded individuals and learn from experts.

**Conclusion**

Staying motivated and accountable on your plant-based journey requires commitment, dedication, and the right strategies. By setting clear goals, tracking your progress, finding a plant-based community, and overcoming common challenges, you'll be well on your way to achieving long-term success on your plant-based journey. Remember to stay positive, focused, and compassionate, and don't be afraid to ask for help along the way. Happy journeying!

# Chapter 12:

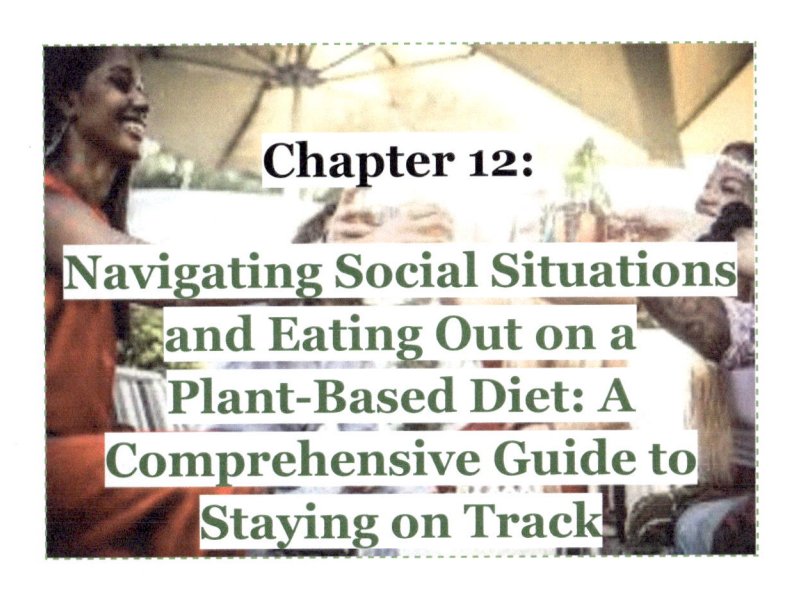

## Navigating Social Situations and Eating Out on a Plant-Based Diet: A Comprehensive Guide to Staying on Track

As a plant-based individual, navigating social situations and eating out can be challenging, but with the right strategies and mindset, you can stay on track and enjoy a variety of delicious and satisfying plant-based options.

**Understanding the Challenges**

Eating out and navigating social situations on a plant-based diet can be challenging for several reasons:

1. Limited options: Many restaurants and social gatherings may not offer plant-based options, making it difficult to find something to eat.
2. Social pressure: You may feel pressure from friends, family, or colleagues to conform to traditional eating habits, making it difficult to stick to your plant-based diet.
3. Lack of knowledge: You may not know how to order plant-based options at restaurants or how to navigate social situations where food is involved.

**Strategies for Navigating Social Situations**

Here are some strategies for navigating social situations on a plant-based diet:

1. Communicate with your host: If you're attending a dinner party or social gathering, let your host know about your plant-based

diet in advance. This will give them time to prepare plant-based options for you.

2. Offer to bring a dish: If you're attending a potluck or social gathering, offer to bring a plant-based dish to share with others. This will ensure that you have something to eat and will also allow others to try plant-based options.

3. Be prepared to answer questions: You may be asked questions about your plant-based diet, such as "Where do you get your protein?" or "Don't you miss cheese?" Be prepared to answer these questions confidently and politely.

4. Find plant-based-friendly social groups: Join plant-based social groups or attend plant-based events to connect with like-minded individuals who share your dietary preferences.

**Strategies for Eating Out**

Here are some strategies for eating out on a plant-based diet:

1. Research plant-based-friendly restaurants: Look for restaurants that offer plant-based options or have a separate plant-based menu. You can use online review sites or social media to find plant-based-friendly restaurants in your area.
2. Ask your server for plant-based options: If you're unsure about what plant-based options are available at a restaurant, ask your server for recommendations. They may be able to suggest plant-based options or offer to modify menu items to make them plant-based.
3. Don't be afraid to ask for modifications: If you see a menu item that can be easily modified to make it plant-based, don't be afraid to ask your server if they can modify it.

For example, you can ask for a veggie burger patty instead of a beef patty.

4. Look for plant-based certifications: Some restaurants may have plant-based certifications, such as the "Plant-Based" symbol or the "Vegan" symbol. These certifications can give you confidence that the restaurant offers plant-based options.

**Plant-Based-Friendly Restaurants and Chains**

Here are some plant-based-friendly restaurants and chains that offer a variety of delicious and satisfying plant-based options:

1. Veggie Grill: A fast-casual chain that offers a variety of plant-based options, including veggie burgers, salads, and bowls.
2. Chipotle Mexican Grill: A fast-casual chain that offers a variety of plant-based options, including burritos, bowls, and tacos.

3. Panera Bread: A bakery-cafe chain that offers a variety of plant-based options, including soups, salads, and sandwiches.
4. Moe's Southwest Grill: A fast-casual chain that offers a variety of plant-based options, including burritos, bowls, and tacos.
5. Jason's Deli: A sandwich chain that offers a variety of plant-based options, including salads, soups, and sandwiches.

## Conclusion

Navigating social situations and eating out on a plant-based diet can be challenging, but with the right strategies and mindset, you can stay on track and enjoy a variety of delicious and satisfying plant-based options. By communicating with your host, offering to bring a dish, being prepared to answer questions, and finding plant-based-friendly social groups and restaurants, you can navigate social situations with confidence and ease. Happy eating!

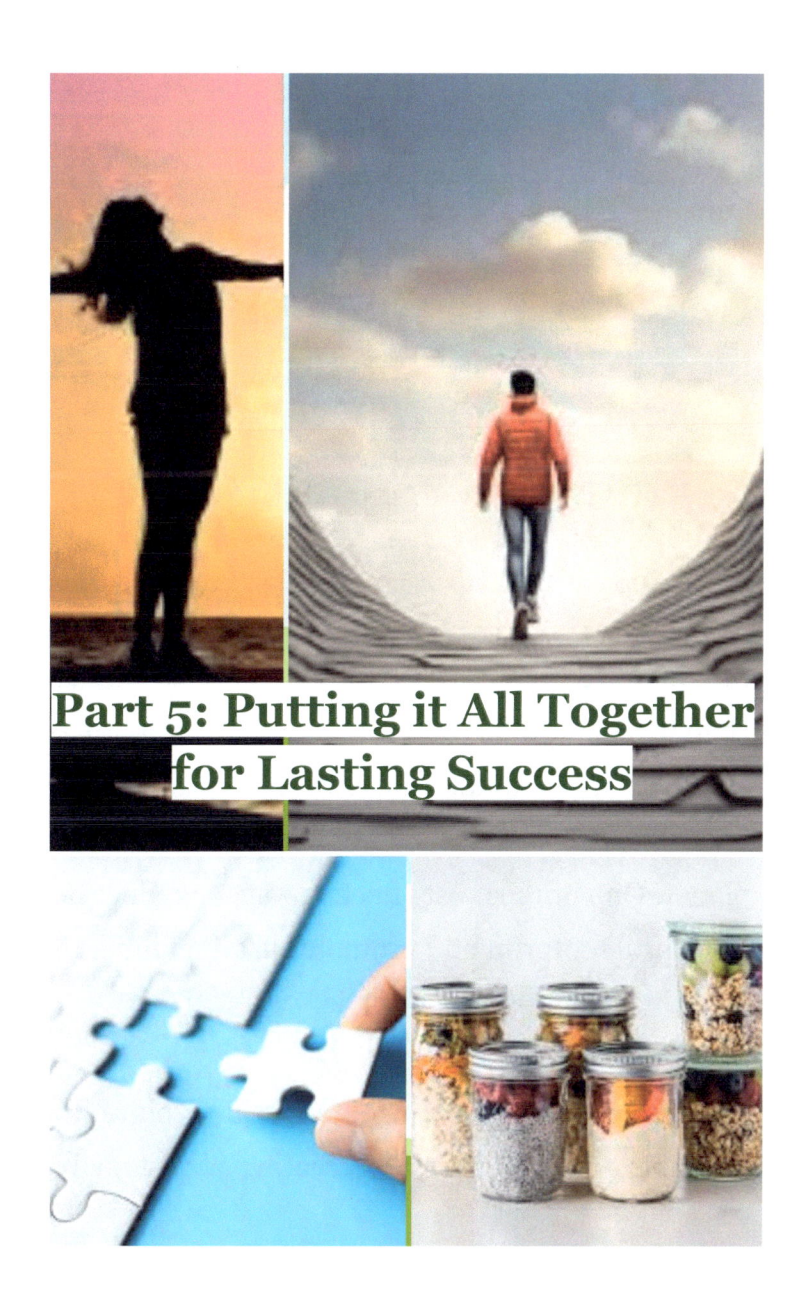

# Part 5: Putting it All Together for Lasting Success

# Chapter 13:

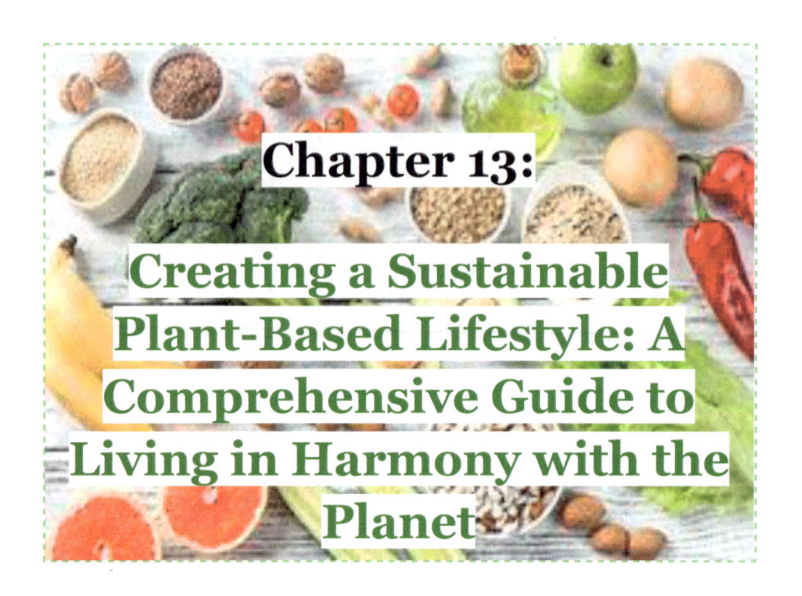

## Creating a Sustainable Plant-Based Lifestyle: A Comprehensive Guide to Living in Harmony with the Planet

As the world grapples with the challenges of climate change, environmental degradation, and social injustice, it's becoming increasingly clear that our lifestyle choices have a profound impact on the planet. One of the most effective ways to reduce our ecological footprint and promote sustainability is by adopting a plant-based lifestyle.

In this comprehensive guide, we'll explore the principles and practices of creating a sustainable plant-based lifestyle that not only nourishes our bodies but also supports the health of the planet.

## Why a Plant-Based Lifestyle is Sustainable

A plant-based lifestyle is inherently sustainable because it:

1. Reduces greenhouse gas emissions: Animal agriculture is a significant contributor to greenhouse gas emissions, deforestation, and water pollution. By choosing plant-based options, we can reduce our carbon footprint and support sustainable agriculture.
2. Conserve water and land: It takes significantly more water and land to produce animal products than plant-based foods. By choosing plant-based options, we can conserve these precious resources and support sustainable agriculture.
3. Promotes biodiversity: Plant-based diets tend to be more diverse and inclusive of a

wide range of fruits, vegetables, whole grains, and legumes. This diversity promotes biodiversity and supports the health of ecosystems.
4. Supports sustainable agriculture: By choosing plant-based options, we can support sustainable agriculture and promote environmentally friendly farming practices.

## Principles of a Sustainable Plant-Based Lifestyle

To create a sustainable plant-based lifestyle, consider the following principles:

1. Whole, minimally processed foods: Focus on whole, minimally processed foods like fruits, vegetables, whole grains, and legumes. These foods tend to be more sustainable and nutritious than processed and packaged foods.
2. Locally sourced and seasonal foods: Choose locally sourced and seasonal foods to reduce

transportation emissions and support local farmers.
3. Reducing food waste: Plan your meals, shop from local farmers, and compost food waste to reduce your ecological footprint.
4. Mindful consumption: Practice mindful consumption by paying attention to your hunger and fullness cues, eating slowly, and savoring your food.

## Practices for a Sustainable Plant-Based Lifestyle

To put these principles into practice, consider the following:

1. Meal planning and prep: Plan your meals, shop for ingredients, and prep your meals in advance to reduce food waste and support sustainable agriculture.
2. Cooking from scratch: Cook from scratch using whole, minimally processed

ingredients to reduce packaging waste and support sustainable agriculture.
3. Reducing single-use plastics: Reduce single-use plastics by choosing reusable bags, containers, and water bottles.
4. Supporting sustainable agriculture: Support sustainable agriculture by choosing organic, locally sourced, and fair-trade options.

## Simple Swaps for a More Sustainable Lifestyle

Here are some simple swaps you can make to create a more sustainable plant-based lifestyle:

1. Swap paper towels for reusable cloths: Switch from paper towels to reusable cloths to reduce paper waste and support sustainable forestry practices.
2. Swap single-use plastics for reusable containers: Switch from single-use plastics to reusable containers to reduce plastic waste and support sustainable agriculture.

3. Swap processed snacks for whole foods: Switch from processed snacks to whole foods like fruits, vegetables, and nuts to reduce packaging waste and support sustainable agriculture.
4. Swap chemical-based cleaning products for natural alternatives: Switch from chemical-based cleaning products to natural alternatives like baking soda and vinegar to reduce toxic waste and support sustainable agriculture.

**Conclusion**

Creating a sustainable plant-based lifestyle is a journey that requires intention, attention, and action. By adopting the principles and practices outlined in this guide, you can create a lifestyle that not only nourishes your body but also supports the health of the planet. Remember, every small step counts and collective action can lead to significant positive change.

# Chapter 14: Mindful Eating and Self-Care for a Healthy Relationship with Food: A Journey of Discovery and Nourishment

In today's fast-paced world, it's easy to get caught up in the hustle and bustle of daily life and forget to prioritize one of the most essential aspects of our well-being: our relationship with food. Mindful eating and self-care are powerful tools that can help us cultivate a healthier, more loving relationship with food and our bodies.

**What is Mindful Eating?**

Mindful eating is the practice of paying attention to our physical and emotional sensations while eating. It's about savoring each bite, noticing the flavors, textures, and aromas, and eating slowly and intentionally. Mindful eating is not just about the food; it's about the experience of eating and the connection we make with our bodies and the world around us.

## Benefits of Mindful Eating

The benefits of mindful eating are numerous and profound. By practicing mindful eating, we can:

1. Develop a healthier relationship with food: Mindful eating helps us let go of unhealthy eating habits, such as emotional eating, bingeing, and restrictive eating.
2. Improve digestion and reduce symptoms of digestive disorders: By eating slowly and intentionally, we can reduce stress and promote healthy digestion.
3. Increase satisfaction and enjoyment of food: Mindful eating helps us appreciate the flavors, textures, and aromas of food, making

mealtime a more enjoyable and satisfying experience.
4. Reduce stress and anxiety: The act of eating can be a source of stress and anxiety, but mindful eating can help us relax and feel more grounded.

**Practicing Mindful Eating**

So, how can we practice mindful eating in our daily lives? Here are some simple yet powerful tips:

1. Start with small, intentional bites: Take small bites and chew slowly, savoring the flavors and textures.
2. Pay attention to your hunger and fullness cues: Eat when you're hungry and stop when you're satisfied, rather than eating out of habit or emotional triggers.
3. Eliminate distractions while eating: Turn off the TV, put away your phone, and eat in a distraction-free environment.

4. Use all of your senses: Notice the colors, textures, and aromas of your food, as well as the sounds and sensations of eating.

**Self-Care and Mindful Eating**

Self-care is an essential aspect of mindful eating. By prioritizing self-care, we can cultivate a more loving and compassionate relationship with our bodies and food. Here are some self-care practices that can support mindful eating:

1. Get enough sleep: Lack of sleep can disrupt our hunger and fullness cues, leading to overeating or poor food choices.
2. Stay hydrated: Drinking plenty of water can help us feel more satisfied and reduce cravings for unhealthy snacks.
3. Engage in regular physical activity: Exercise can help us feel more grounded and connected to our bodies, making it easier to make healthy food choices.

4. Practice stress-reducing techniques: Stress can trigger emotional eating and poor food choices. Practicing stress-reducing techniques like meditation, deep breathing, or yoga can help us feel more calm and centered.

**Creating a Self-Care Practice**

Creating a self-care practice that supports mindful eating can be simple and enjoyable. Here are some ideas to get you started:

1. Schedule self-care time into your daily routine: Set aside time each day for activities that nourish your mind, body, and spirit.
2. Try journaling or reflection: Writing down your thoughts, feelings, and insights can help you process your emotions and develop a greater awareness of your relationship with food.

3. Experiment with different self-care activities: Try different activities like meditation, yoga, or walking to find what works best for you.
4. Make self-care a non-negotiable part of your daily routine: Prioritize self-care and make it a non-negotiable part of your daily routine.

**Final Thoughts**

Mindful eating and self-care are powerful tools that can help us cultivate a healthier, more loving relationship with food and our bodies. By practicing mindful eating and prioritizing self-care, we can develop a greater awareness of our thoughts, feelings, and physical sensations, making it easier to make healthy food choices and cultivate a positive body image. Remember, the journey to mindful eating and self-care is a journey of discovery and nourishment. Be patient, kind, and compassionate with yourself as you explore this journey, and remember to celebrate your successes along the way.

# Chapter 15:

## Maintaining Momentum and Celebrating Your Successes: The Key to Long-Term Success on Your Plant-Based Journey

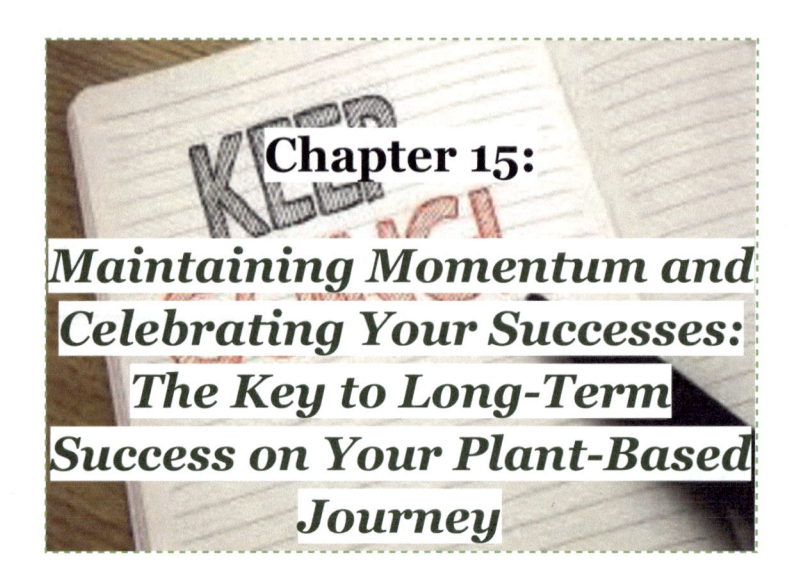

Congratulations on taking the first step towards a healthier, more compassionate lifestyle! As you continue on your plant-based journey, it's essential to maintain momentum and celebrate your successes along the way. In this comprehensive guide, we'll explore the strategies and techniques you need to stay motivated, overcome obstacles, and celebrate your achievements.

**Why Maintaining Momentum is Crucial**

Maintaining momentum is crucial to long-term success on your plant-based journey. Here are just a few reasons why:

1. Prevents burnout: When you're constantly pushing yourself to make changes, it's easy to burn out. Maintaining momentum helps you avoid burnout and stay motivated.
2. Helps you overcome obstacles: Life is full of obstacles, and maintaining momentum helps you overcome them. Whether it's a busy schedule, lack of motivation, or temptation, maintaining momentum helps you stay on track.
3. Boosts confidence: Celebrating your successes and maintaining momentum boosts your confidence and self-esteem. When you see the progress you're making, you'll feel more motivated to continue.
4. Supports long-term success: Maintaining momentum is essential to long-term success on your plant-based journey. When you stay

motivated and focused, you're more likely to achieve your goals and maintain a healthy, balanced lifestyle.

**Strategies for Maintaining Momentum**

Here are some strategies for maintaining momentum on your plant-based journey:

1. Set realistic goals: Setting realistic goals helps you stay motivated and focused. Break down your long-term goals into smaller, achievable milestones.
2. Create a support network: Surround yourself with people who support and encourage you. Join online communities, attend plant-based events, or find a plant-based buddy.
3. Track your progress: Tracking your progress helps you stay motivated and see the progress you're making. Use a food diary, mobile app, or spreadsheet to track your progress.

4. Celebrate your successes: Celebrating your successes is essential to maintaining momentum. Treat yourself to something special, share your achievements with friends and family, or write about your successes in a journal.
5. Stay positive and focused: Stay positive and focused by surrounding yourself with inspiring stories, motivational quotes, and uplifting music.

**Techniques for Overcoming Obstacles**

Here are some techniques for overcoming obstacles on your plant-based journey:

1. Identify your triggers: Identify your triggers and develop strategies to overcome them. Whether it's stress, boredom, or temptation, having a plan in place helps you stay on track.

2. Find healthy alternatives: Find healthy alternatives to your favorite comfort foods or treats. Whether it's a plant-based version of your favorite dessert or a healthy snack, having alternatives helps you stay on track.
3. Practice self-care: Practice self-care by getting enough sleep, exercising regularly, and taking time for relaxation and stress relief.
4. Seek support: Seek support from friends, family, or a plant-based community. Having a support network helps you stay motivated and overcome obstacles.
5. Focus on progress, not perfection: Focus on progress, not perfection. Remember that setbacks are a normal part of the journey, and don't be too hard on yourself when you slip up.

## Celebrating Your Successes

Celebrating your successes is essential to maintaining momentum and staying motivated on your plant-based journey. Here are some ways to celebrate your successes:

1. Treat yourself to something special: Treat yourself to something special, like a plant-based dessert or a new cookbook.
2. Share your achievements with friends and family: Share your achievements with friends and family, and ask them to support and encourage you on your journey.
3. Write about your successes in a journal: Write about your successes in a journal, and reflect on how far you've come.
4. Take progress photos: Take progress photos, and celebrate your physical and emotional transformations.
5. Host a plant-based dinner party: Host a plant-based dinner party, and share your

favorite plant-based dishes with friends and family.

**Final Thoughts**

Maintaining momentum and celebrating your successes are essential to long-term success on your plant-based journey. By setting realistic goals, creating a support network, tracking your progress, and celebrating your successes, you'll stay motivated and focused on your goals. Remember to stay positive, focused, and compassionate, and don't be too hard on yourself when you slip up. Congratulations on taking the first step towards a healthier, more compassionate lifestyle!

# Conclusion

## *Congratulations on Completing the Plant-Based Diet for Weight Loss Journey!*

Dear friend, we are beyond thrilled to congratulate you on completing the plant-based diet for weight loss journey! This is a remarkable achievement, and we couldn't be prouder of you.

**Your Journey, Your Success**

Over the past few weeks, you've worked tirelessly to transform your relationship with food and your body. You've learned how to nourish your body with whole, plant-based foods, and you've discovered the incredible benefits of this lifestyle. Your hard work and dedication have paid off, and you should be incredibly proud of yourself.

**The Power of Plant-Based Living**

As you've learned throughout this journey, plant-based living is not just a diet – it's a lifestyle. It's a way of living that promotes overall health, wellness, and sustainability. By choosing whole, plant-based foods, you're not only transforming your health but also contributing to a more compassionate and environmentally friendly world.

**Your Weight Loss Success**

We know that weight loss was a significant goal for you on this journey, and we're thrilled to see that you've achieved success in this area. Your hard work and dedication to healthy eating and regular physical activity have paid off, and you should be incredibly proud of yourself.

**Beyond Weight Loss: The Many Benefits of Plant-Based Living**

While weight loss is an incredible achievement, it's just one of the many benefits of plant-based living. As you've learned throughout this journey, a well-planned plant-based diet can help:

- Lower cholesterol and blood pressure
- Improve blood sugar control
- Reduce the risk of chronic diseases like heart disease, type 2 diabetes, and certain types of cancer
- Support healthy weight management
- Improve mental health and mood
- Support healthy digestion and gut health

**What's Next?**

Now that you've completed the plant-based diet for weight loss journey, you might be wondering what's next. Here are a few suggestions to help you continue on your path to optimal health and wellness:

- Continue to explore new plant-based recipes and ingredients to keep your diet interesting and varied.
- Incorporate physical activity into your daily routine, such as walking, jogging, yoga, or weightlifting.
- Stay connected with like-minded individuals through online communities or local plant-based groups.
- Continue to educate yourself on the benefits of plant-based living and share your knowledge with others.

**Celebrating Your Success**

We want to celebrate your success with you! Take some time to reflect on your journey and all that you've accomplished. Treat yourself to a special plant-based meal or dessert, and share your success with friends and family.

**You Did It!**

Once again, congratulations on completing the plant-based diet for weight loss journey! You should be incredibly proud of yourself and all that you've accomplished. Remember, this is just the beginning of your journey to optimal health and wellness. Keep shining, and we'll be cheering you on every step of the way!

# Next Steps and Continued Support: Empowering Your Ongoing Plant-Based Journey

Congratulations on completing the plant-based diet for the weight loss journey! As you celebrate your successes and reflect on your progress, it's essential to consider your next steps and how you'll continue to support your plant-based lifestyle.

**Why Ongoing Support is Crucial**

Embarking on a plant-based journey can be a significant life change, and it's essential to have ongoing support to ensure long-term success. Here are just a few reasons why ongoing support is crucial:

1. Accountability: Having a support system in place helps you stay accountable and

motivated, even when faced with challenges or setbacks.
2. Guidance and advice: Ongoing support provides you with access to guidance and advice from experienced professionals, helping you navigate any obstacles or concerns that may arise.
3. Community connection: Connecting with like-minded individuals through ongoing support helps you feel part of a community, reducing feelings of isolation and increasing motivation.
4. Continued education: Ongoing support provides you with access to continued education and resources, helping you stay up-to-date on the latest plant-based research, recipes, and lifestyle tips.

**Next Steps for Your Plant-Based Journey**

As you move forward on your plant-based journey, here are some next steps to consider:

1. Set new goals and challenges: Setting new goals and challenges helps you stay motivated and focused, ensuring continued progress and success.
2. Explore new recipes and ingredients: Continuously exploring new recipes and ingredients helps keep your diet interesting and varied, reducing the risk of boredom or burnout.
3. Incorporate physical activity and self-care: Regular physical activity and self-care are essential for overall health and wellness. Incorporate activities like yoga, walking, or meditation into your daily routine.
4. Stay connected with the plant-based community: Connecting with like-minded individuals through online forums, social media groups, or local plant-based meetups helps you feel part of a community and stay motivated.

**Continued Support Options**

To support your ongoing plant-based journey, consider the following continued support options:

1. Online communities and forums: Join online communities and forums dedicated to plant-based living, providing access to guidance, advice, and support from experienced professionals and like-minded individuals.
2. Plant-based coaches or mentors: Work with a plant-based coach or mentor who can provide personalized guidance, support, and accountability.
3. Local plant-based meetups and events: Attend local plant-based meetups and events, providing opportunities to connect with like-minded individuals and stay motivated.
4. Plant-based retreats and workshops: Consider attending plant-based retreats and workshops, offering immersive experiences

and opportunities to learn from experienced professionals.

## Conclusion

Congratulations again on completing the plant-based diet for weight loss journey! As you move forward on your plant-based journey, remember that ongoing support is crucial for long-term success. By setting new goals and challenges, exploring new recipes and ingredients, incorporating physical activity and self-care, and staying connected with the plant-based community, you'll be empowered to continue thriving on your plant-based journey.

# Appendix

## *Plant-Based Resources and Recommendations: A Comprehensive Guide to Supporting Your Plant-Based Lifestyle*

As you continue on your plant-based journey, it's essential to have access to reliable resources and recommendations to support your lifestyle. In this comprehensive guide, we'll explore the best plant-based resources and recommendations, covering everything from cookbooks and documentaries to online communities and local restaurants.

**Online Resources**

The internet is a treasure trove of plant-based resources, offering a wealth of information, inspiration, and support. Here are some of the best online resources to support your plant-based lifestyle:

1. Websites and Blogs:
- Oh, She Glows: A popular plant-based blog featuring recipes, lifestyle tips, and product reviews.
- The Full Helping: A comprehensive plant-based resource offering recipes, cooking tips, and lifestyle advice.
- Plant-Based News: A leading online news source dedicated to plant-based living, featuring the latest news, trends, and product reviews.
2. Social Media:
- Instagram: Follow plant-based influencers and bloggers like @ohsheglows, @thefullhelping, and @plantbasednews for inspiration, recipes, and lifestyle tips.
- Facebook: Join plant-based groups like Plant-Based Living, Vegan Support Group,

and Plant-Based Recipes for support, advice, and community connection.

3. Online Communities:
- Plant-Based Forum: A comprehensive online forum dedicated to plant-based living, featuring discussions, recipes, and lifestyle advice.
- Vegan Forum: A popular online community for vegans, offering support, advice, and resources for plant-based living.

**Cookbooks and Recipe Resources**

Cookbooks and recipe resources are essential for any plant-based kitchen. Here are some of the best cookbooks and recipe resources to support your plant-based lifestyle:

1. Cookbooks:
→ "The Oh She Glows Cookbook" by Angela Liddon: A comprehensive plant-based cookbook featuring over 100 recipes.

- → "Thrive" by Brendan Brazier: A plant-based cookbook focused on high-performance nutrition and wellness.
- → "The Plant Paradox Cookbook" by Dr. Steven Gundry: A plant-based cookbook featuring over 100 recipes and focused on gut health and wellness.

2. Recipe Websites:
- Oh, She Glows: A popular plant-based recipe website featuring over 500 recipes.
- The Full Helping: A comprehensive plant-based recipe website featuring a wide range of recipes and cooking tips.
- Plant-Based Recipes: A popular recipe website featuring a wide range of plant-based recipes and cooking tips.

**Documentaries and Films**

Documentaries and films are a great way to learn more about plant-based living and the benefits of a plant-based lifestyle. Here are some of the best documentaries and films to support your plant-based lifestyle:

1. Documentaries:
   - "What the Health" (2017): A documentary exploring the link between diet and disease, featuring interviews with leading health experts.
   - "Forks Over Knives" (2011): A documentary exploring the benefits of a plant-based diet, featuring interviews with leading health experts.
   - "Cowspiracy" (2014): A documentary exploring the environmental impact of animal agriculture, featuring interviews with leading environmental experts.
2. Films:
   - "PlantPure Nation" (2015): A film exploring the benefits of a plant-based diet, featuring interviews with leading health experts.
   - "The Game Changers" (2018): A film exploring the benefits of a plant-based diet

for athletes and fitness enthusiasts, featuring interviews with leading athletes and health experts.

## Local Resources and Recommendations

In addition to online resources, it's essential to have access to local resources and recommendations to support your plant-based lifestyle. Here are some local resources and recommendations to consider:

1. Local Health Food Stores:
- Visit local health food stores in your area for plant-based groceries, supplements, and lifestyle products.
2. Plant-Based Restaurants and Cafes:
- Visit local plant-based restaurants and cafes for delicious and inspiring plant-based meals.
3. Local Farmers Markets:
- Visit local farmers markets for fresh, seasonal produce and plant-based products.
4. Plant-Based Meetups and Events:

- Attend local plant-based meetups and events for support, advice, and community connection.

**Mobile Apps**
1. Happy Cow: A popular mobile app featuring plant-based restaurant and store listings, as well as recipes and lifestyle tips.
2. Is It Vegan?: A mobile app helping users identify vegan-friendly products and ingredients.
3. Plant-Based Diet: A mobile app providing plant-based recipes, meal planning, and lifestyle tips.

**Podcasts**
1. The Plant-Based Podcast: A popular podcast exploring plant-based living, featuring interviews with leading health experts and thought leaders.

2. The Vegan Podcast: A podcast dedicated to vegan living, featuring interviews with leading vegan experts and thought leaders.
3. The Plant Paradox Podcast: A podcast exploring the benefits of plant-based living, featuring interviews with leading health experts and thought leaders.

**Books**

1. "The Plant Paradox" by Dr. Steven Gundry: A book exploring the benefits of plant-based living, focusing on gut health and wellness.
2. "The Blue Zones" by Dan Buettner: A book exploring the world's longest-lived communities, highlighting the importance of plant-based living.
3. "How Not to Die" by Dr. Michael Greger: A book exploring the benefits of plant-based living, focusing on disease prevention and reversal.

**Online Courses and Programs**
1. Plant-Based Nutrition Certification Program: A comprehensive online program offering certification in plant-based nutrition.
2. Vegan Nutrition Course: An online course exploring vegan nutrition, featuring lessons and lectures from leading health experts.
3. Plant-Based Cooking Course: An online course teaching plant-based cooking techniques and recipes.

**Conclusion**

In conclusion, there are many amazing plant-based resources and recommendations available to support your plant-based lifestyle. From online resources and cookbooks to documentaries and local recommendations, there's something for everyone. Remember to always stay curious, keep learning, and have fun exploring the world of plant-based living!

# *Meal Planning Templates and Worksheets: A Comprehensive Guide to Planning Delicious and Healthy Plant-Based Meals*

Meal planning is an essential part of maintaining a healthy and balanced plant-based diet. It helps you save time, reduce food waste, and ensure that you're getting all the nutrients your body needs. In this guide, we'll explore the benefits of meal planning, provide you with customizable meal planning templates and worksheets, and offer tips and tricks for planning delicious and healthy plant-based meals.

**Benefits of Meal Planning**

Meal planning offers numerous benefits, including:

1. Saves time: Meal planning helps you save time during the week when you're busy with work, school, or other activities. By planning your meals, you can quickly and easily prepare healthy meals without having to spend hours thinking about what to cook.
2. Reduces food waste: Meal planning helps you avoid buying too much food that may go to waste. By planning your meals, you can make a grocery list and stick to it, reducing food waste and saving you money.
3. Ensures healthy eating: Meal planning helps you ensure that you're getting all the nutrients your body needs. By planning your meals, you can make sure that you're including a variety of fruits, vegetables, whole grains, and plant-based protein sources in your diet.
4. Supports weight loss: Meal planning can help support weight loss by ensuring that you're eating healthy, portion-controlled meals. By planning your meals, you can

avoid relying on fast food or processed snacks that are high in calories and low in nutrients.

## Meal Planning Templates and Worksheets

To help you get started with meal planning, we've provided you with customizable meal planning templates and worksheets. These templates and worksheets can be downloaded and printed, or filled out digitally.

1. Weekly Meal Planning Template: This template provides a space for you to plan out your meals for the week. It includes sections for breakfast, lunch, dinner, and snacks, as well as a space for you to note down your grocery list.
2. Daily Meal Planning Worksheet: This worksheet provides a space for you to plan out your meals for the day. It includes sections for breakfast, lunch, dinner, and

snacks, as well as a space for you to note down your water intake and physical activity.
3. Grocery List Template: This template provides a space for you to note down your grocery list. It includes sections for produce, grains, protein sources, and pantry staples.
4. Meal Planning Calendar: This calendar provides a space for you to plan out your meals for the month. It includes sections for each day of the month, as well as a space for you to note down your grocery list and meal planning notes.

**Tips and Tricks for Meal Planning**

Here are some tips and tricks for meal planning that you may find helpful:

1. Start small: If you're new to meal planning, start small by planning out your meals for a few days or a week. As you get more comfortable with meal planning, you can

start planning out your meals for longer periods.

2. Be flexible: Meal planning is not a one-size-fits-all approach. Be flexible and willing to make changes to your meal plan as needed.

3. Include a variety of foods: Make sure to include a variety of foods in your meal plan, including fruits, vegetables, whole grains, and plant-based protein sources.

4. Make a grocery list: Make a grocery list based on your meal plan and stick to it. This will help you avoid buying unnecessary items and reduce food waste.

5. Cook in bulk: Cooking in bulk can save you time and money. Consider cooking large batches of rice, beans, or grains and using them throughout the week in different meals.

## Conclusion

Meal planning is an essential part of maintaining a healthy and balanced plant-based diet. By using the meal planning templates and worksheets provided in this guide, you can plan delicious and healthy plant-based meals that meet your nutritional needs and support your overall health and well-being. Remember to be flexible, include a variety of foods, make a grocery list, and cook in bulk to make meal planning easier and more efficient. Happy meal planning!

Here are some templates and worksheets for meal planning:

## Weekly Meal Planning Template

| DAY | B/FAST | LUNCH | DINNER | SNACK |
|---|---|---|---|---|
| MON | | | | |
| TUE | | | | |
| WED | | | | |
| THU | | | | |

| | | | | |
|---|---|---|---|---|
| FRI | | | | |
| SAT | | | | |
| SUN | | | | |

## Daily Meal Planning Worksheet

| MEAL | FOOD | PORTION SIZE | CALORIES |
|---|---|---|---|
| B/FAST | | | |
| LUNCH | | | |
| DINNER | | | |
| SNACK | | | |

## Grocery List Template

| CATEGORY | ITEM | QUANTITY |
|---|---|---|
| PRODUCE | | |
| GRAINS | | |
| PROTEIN | | |
| PANTRY | | |
| SNACKS | | |

## Meal Planning Calendar

| WEEK | MON | TUE | WED | THU | FRI | SAT | SUN |
|---|---|---|---|---|---|---|---|
| 1 | | | | | | | |
| 2 | | | | | | | |
| 3 | | | | | | | |
| 4 | | | | | | | |

## Plant-Based Meal Planning Worksheet

| MEAL | PLANT BASED PROTEIN | VEGETABLES | WHOLE GRAIN | HEALTHY FATS |
|---|---|---|---|---|
| B/FAST | | | | |
| LUNCH | | | | |
| DINNER | | | | |
| SNACKS | | | | |

## Meal Planning Reflection Worksheet

| DAY | MEAL | HOW DID I FEEL? | WHAT DID I LEARN? | WHAT WOULD I CHANGE? |
|---|---|---|---|---|
| | | | | |

| | | | | |
|---|---|---|---|---|
| MON | | | | |
| TUE | | | | |
| WED | | | | |
| THU | | | | |
| FRI | | | | |
| SAT | | | | |
| SUN | | | | |

**Here are the rest of the templates and worksheets:**

**Meal Planning Budget Worksheet**

| CATEGORY | BUDGETED AMOUNT | ACTUAL SPEND |
|---|---|---|
| PRODUCE | | |
| GRAIN | | |
| PROTEIN | | |
| PANTRY | | |
| TOTAL | | |

## Meal Planning Grocery List Worksheet

| STORE | ITEM | QUANTITY | PRICE |
|-------|------|----------|-------|
|       |      |          |       |
|       |      |          |       |
|       |      |          |       |

## Meal Planning Recipe Worksheet

| RECIPE | INGREDIENTS | INSTRUCTIONS | NUTRITION INFO |
|--------|-------------|--------------|----------------|
|        |             |              |                |
|        |             |              |                |
|        |             |              |                |

## Meal Planning Meal Prep Worksheet

| MEAL | PREP TIME | COOK TIME | TOTAL TIME |
|------|-----------|-----------|------------|
|      |           |           |            |

|  |  |  |  |
|--|--|--|--|
|  |  |  |  |

## Meal Planning Leftovers Worksheet

| MEAL | LEFTOVERS | REHEATING INSTRUCTION |
|------|-----------|----------------------|
|      |           |                      |
|      |           |                      |
|      |           |                      |

These templates and worksheets are designed to help you plan and organize your meals, make grocery lists, and stay within your budget. You can print them out or fill them out digitally, and customize them to fit your needs.

I hope these templates and worksheets are helpful! Let me know if you have any questions or need further assistance.

# Plant-Based Nutrition Glossary: Unlocking the Secrets of a Healthy and Balanced Plant-Based Diet

As you embark on your plant-based journey, it's essential to understand the language of plant-based nutrition. This comprehensive glossary will guide you through the world of plant-based nutrition, explaining key terms, concepts, and nutrients in simple and clear terms.

**Antioxidants**

Antioxidants are compounds that help protect cells from damage caused by free radicals. Plant-based foods rich in antioxidants include berries, leafy greens, and other fruits and vegetables.

**Bioavailability**

Bioavailability refers to the extent to which the body can absorb and utilize nutrients from food. Plant-based foods with high bioavailability include leafy greens, beans, and lentils.

**Carotenoids**
Carotenoids are a group of pigments found in plant-based foods, such as sweet potatoes, carrots, and dark leafy greens. They convert to vitamin A in the body and support healthy vision, immune function, and skin health.

**Complete Protein**
A complete protein is a protein that contains all nine essential amino acids that the body cannot produce on its own. Plant-based complete proteins include quinoa, chia seeds, and hemp seeds.

**Dietary Fiber**
Dietary fiber is a type of carbohydrate found in plant-based foods, such as fruits, vegetables, whole

grains, and legumes. It supports healthy digestion, satiety, and blood sugar control.

**Essential Fatty Acids (EFAs)**
EFAs are a type of fatty acid that the body cannot produce on its own. Plant-based sources of EFAs include chia seeds, flaxseeds, and walnuts.

**Flavonoids**
Flavonoids are a group of plant compounds that support healthy heart function, blood pressure, and cognitive function. Plant-based foods rich in flavonoids include berries, apples, and onions.

**Free Radicals**
Free radicals are unstable molecules that can cause oxidative stress and damage to cells. Plant-based foods rich in antioxidants, such as berries and leafy greens, can help neutralize free radicals.

**Glycemic Index (GI)**

The GI is a measure of how quickly a food raises blood sugar levels. Plant-based foods with a low GI include whole grains, fruits, and vegetables.

**Hydrogenation**
Hydrogenation is a process that converts unsaturated fats into saturated fats, making them more solid and increasing their shelf life. Plant-based foods that are often hydrogenated include margarine and vegetable shortening.

**Isothiocyanates**
Isothiocyanates are a group of plant compounds that support healthy detoxification and cancer prevention. Plant-based foods rich in isothiocyanates include broccoli, cauliflower, and kale.

**Lectins**
Lectins are a type of protein found in plant-based foods, such as beans, grains, and nightshades. They

can cause inflammation and digestive issues in some individuals.

## Lignans

Lignans are a group of plant compounds that support healthy hormone balance and cancer prevention. Plant-based foods rich in lignans include flaxseeds, chia seeds, and sesame seeds.

## Macronutrients

Macronutrients are the three main categories of nutrients: carbohydrates, protein, and fat. Plant-based foods provide a balanced mix of macronutrients.

## Micronutrients

Micronutrients are vitamins and minerals that support healthy growth and development. Plant-based foods provide a rich source of micronutrients, including vitamins A, C, and E, and minerals like potassium and iron.

## Omega-3 Fatty Acids

Omega-3 fatty acids are a type of EFA that supports healthy heart function and brain development. Plant-based sources of omega-3s include chia seeds, flaxseeds, and walnuts.

## Oxidative Stress

Oxidative stress occurs when the body's antioxidant defenses are overwhelmed by free radicals. Plant-based foods rich in antioxidants, such as berries and leafy greens, can help reduce oxidative stress.

## Phytochemicals

Phytochemicals are a group of plant compounds that support healthy growth and development. Plant-based foods rich in phytochemicals include fruits, vegetables, whole grains, and legumes.

## Polyphenols

Polyphenols are a group of plant compounds that support healthy heart function, cognitive function, and cancer prevention. Plant-based foods rich in polyphenols include berries, apples, and onions.

**Probiotics**

Probiotics are beneficial bacteria that support healthy gut function and immune system function. Plant-based sources of probiotics include fermented foods like kimchi, sauerkraut, and miso.

**Protein**

Protein is a macronutrient that supports healthy growth and development. Plant-based sources of protein include beans, lentils, tofu, tempeh, and seitan.

**Saturated Fat**

Saturated fat is a type of fat that can raise cholesterol levels and increase the risk of heart disease. Plant-based sources of saturated fat include coconut oil, palm oil, and palm kernel oil.

## Tannins

Tannins are a group of plant compounds that can bind to proteins and carbohydrates, making them less available for absorption. Plant-based foods rich in tannins include tea, coffee, and dark chocolate.

## Trans Fat

Trans fat is a type of unsaturated fat that can raise cholesterol levels and increase the risk of heart disease. Plant-based sources of trans fat include partially hydrogenated oils.

## Unsaturated Fat

Unsaturated fat is a type of fat that can help lower cholesterol levels and reduce the risk of heart disease. Plant-based sources of unsaturated fat include nuts, seeds, avocados, and olive oil.

## Vegan

Vegan refers to a diet that excludes all animal products, including meat, dairy, eggs, and honey.

**Vegetarian**

Vegetarian refers to a diet that excludes meat, fish, and poultry, but may include dairy and eggs.

**Vitamin**

Vitamin refers to a nutrient that is essential for healthy growth and development. Plant-based sources of vitamins include fruits, vegetables, whole grains, and legumes.

**Whole Food**

Whole food refers to a food that is unprocessed and unrefined, containing all of its natural nutrients and fiber. Plant-based whole foods include fruits, vegetables, whole grains, and legumes.

**Zenosterols**

Zenosterols are a group of plant compounds that can help lower cholesterol levels and reduce the risk of heart disease. Plant-based foods rich in zenosterols include rice bran, wheat germ, and sesame seeds.

By understanding these key terms and concepts, you'll be better equipped to navigate the world of plant-based nutrition and make informed choices about the foods you eat. Remember to always consult with a healthcare professional or registered dietitian for personalized nutrition advice.